GUT INSTINCT

Transform
your life and health
with the power
of your gut.

The information provided in this book is designed to provide helpful information on the subjects discussed and are for informational purposes only. This book is not meant to be used, nor should it be used, to diagnose or treat any medical condition. For diagnosis or treatment of any medical problem, consult your own physician. The publisher and author or anyone else associated with this book, are not responsible for any specific health or allergy needs that may require medical supervision and are not liable for any damages or negative consequences from any treatment, action, application, or preparation, to any person reading or following the information in this book. References are provided for informational purposes only and do not constitute endorsement of any websites or other sources. Readers should be aware that the websites listed in this book may change.

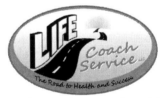
Cover designer: Jesse Hale, Baysidesigns.biz
Editor: Ashley Sprague
Illustrator: Reuel Cornelison

ISBN: 978-0-9976764-0-2

About the Author

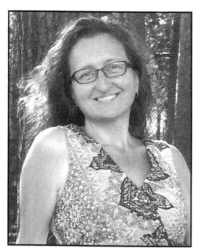

Carolyn O'Byrne

Carolyn O'Byrne, CHT, author of ***Gut Instinct, Transform Your Life and Health with the Power of Your Gut*** is a colon hydrotherapist and a life coach. Her passion is to reach even more people by using this book as another way to help others who are desiring change in their lives. She is there to show them how to transform their future and to direct them to success, to health, and to a positive outlook on life.

Throughout her years of interest in true health and wellness, she has studied and applied to her own life these many different modalities. Her insight has also enabled her to help numerous others on their journey to health through her business, Life Coach Service, LLC. Her mission is to steer those who want results in the direction of good health, both emotionally and physically.

Blessings on your journey to health. Carolyn O'Byrne 3/17

Contents

Preface

Drivers, I am on your side, and my goal is to help you and your loved ones to achieve excellent health. With this information, let me support you in boosting your health into overdrive, a destination that you only have dreamed about. It is very possible, and I am going to present to you some tools for doing it right. Anyone can just read this information, but I am writing this book for those of you out there who are the take-charge, go-getter kind of people who want better health but until now have not known how to achieve it.

Because of my dedication to my family and to you, I bring you this simple, no-nonsense, common-sense book that addresses the connection and importance of gut health to overall health. I am hoping to help the hard-working individuals reading this to be aware of this important information and to be able to apply it to their lives. Those of you who are committed to change will also get some great ideas on how to prepare your own food.

You spend time and money to maintain your truck. YOU are more important than your truck. If you are not healthy, that truck is not going anywhere. Put your health first. This book is not only for you, driver, it is for your friends and your family. How much more can you enjoy each other when you are all experiencing good health? Put these ideas into practice. Make them part of your lives, and you will all see the benefit.

Gratitude

I want to thank God for the opportunity to write this book. My intention is to help others to achieve their best health and highest good. I want to thank the following people: my wonderful husband, whom I love dearly, and who works so hard pushing that truck down the road in order to provide for his family and who has been there for me and supported me as my cheerleader and best friend; my children, whom I also love

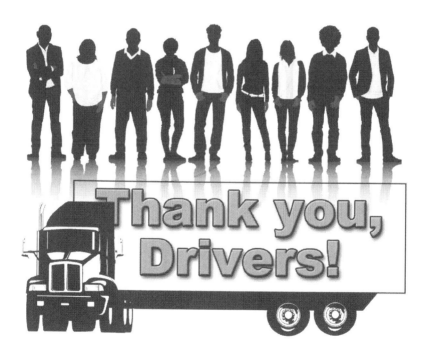

dearly. You are my inspiration to learn more every day. Thank you for putting up with my spending long hours in my work space; Tammy and Sandy for untold amounts of talent, insight, motivation, and encouragement; my lovely and brilliant editor Ashley Sprague; Jesse and Stephanie Hale, my friends and book cover designer; Reuel Cornelison for so much direction and kindness; Vicki Haygood for your great talent; Donna and Allen Smith with Ask the Trucker and Trucking Social Media, who have provided thoughtful guidance along the way; truckers Jimmy Ardis for giving me inspiration, Jeannie Lennox, Idella Hanson, Sandi Talbott, Tom Kyrk, and Jimmy Kelley for your direction and enthusiasm while on the road. Thank you to all the drivers out there whom I have and have not met but hope to. You keep this country rolling. I have the deepest gratitude for you all. Blessings.

My Story, the Secret is Out

As a child I was always fascinated with nature and stayed in the woods as much as possible, tasting and exploring trees, weeds, and berries. It is a wonder that I survived. These strong curiosities led me to an interest in herbalism. After becoming an adult, I studied and read everything that I could on the subject, not knowing how much it would have an impact on my life and the lives of others. This different way of thinking kept my mind open to many other alternative interests in healing. Through many serious, and not so serious, health challenges of family, friends, and sometimes strangers, I gained much knowledge, wisdom, and seemingly common sense on the natural way to health.

As long as I can remember back through childhood, I recall having bowel trouble. Through the years of growing up, I just accepted that this was just the way it was. By the time I was about twenty years old, I was in a mess. I went to the doctor, who informed me of my unhealthy state. I had severe acid reflux (I could have told him that.), irritable bowel syndrome, spastic colon, constipation, high triglycerides and cholesterol, acne, and I was overweight. At twenty??? How could this be? They put me on three different medications and told me to come back often to keep a check on things. I asked them, "How long do I have to take this medication?" The answer was, "The rest of your life."

Well, looking back I can now see very clearly what the problem was. You see even though I ran around the woods as a child experimenting with nature, at meal time we ate the SAD (Standard American Diet) way. This is NOT what our bodies are designed to run on. Think of your truck. If you put any other kind of fuel in it than what was designed for it, will it run??? Of course not! We are much more complicated than that. We are designed to eat only a certain way, and when that way is accomplished, we will run like a charm.

After that doctor appointment when I realized that my health was not good, I searched here and there and put my new knowledge to use, and little by little, my health improved. Within one year of that appointment, I was off all medications. I have NEVER taken them again! Now when I go for a checkup, they usually check my results two or three times because they don't believe it. They always tell me the test results look like a teenager's.

The first nine months of one of my children's life was spent in and out of the doctor's office. It seemed like this ear infection would hit every other Wednesday. She would be prescribed a ten day antibiotic and fourteen days later, we were back at the doctor. During this time we were visiting a friend on the other side of the country, and here we go again, screaming ear pain for hours. Since we were a very long way from home, and it was at night, the emergency room was our only choice. And again, another antibiotic. I'D HAD ENOUGH! I was determined to figure this out. When we got back home, I searched high and low for what to do for this child. Obviously what we had been doing wasn't working. I found something called ear oil at the local health food store and tried it. We have never had another ear infection again. What was in it? Olive oil and garlic, nothing else.

The most explosive and memorable shove into an even more natural way of thinking was when my youngest child had a life-threatening illness that was predicted to be fatal. *IF* she survived, her quality of life would not be good. Because of the significant amount of antibiotics and a long list of other medications she'd been prescribed, her digestive system was completely shot. She was in misery from the inside out with extreme digestive issues including discomfort and lack of nutrient absorption. She also had very unpleasant and downright painful bouts of terror in the bathroom. Severe eczema, rashes, dry scaly skin, and the cracked, bleeding, painful boo boo's on her hands and feet plagued her little body. Creams and medications did nothing. The doctors didn't even know what to do. It was up to me to figure this mystery out. Nothing was stopping this mommy on a quest. In my hundreds of hours of research and a tip from a friend, I discovered more and more information on the health and workings of the digestive system. THAT WAS IT!!! So I went back to school to learn about this extremely interesting and important topic that is so under-recognized.

Immediately we started putting into action what I was learning. It was like a magical wonder. You mean all this time and all this suffering for nothing? Why didn't doctors tell me this? Why did I have to dig to the depths and even go back to school to learn things that should be common knowledge or at least told to us by people we pay to help us to stay healthy?

She was in NO more pain. Her eczema and rashes were gone, and she had no more agony in the bathroom. All this with no creams and no medications. The whole family was benefiting from this "new-found knowledge" and life-changing way of living. Oh boy, did it help out on the road! My husband, a second generation truck driver, lost weight. He said that when he would jump in and out of the truck there were no more achy joints. He had more energy, clearer thinking, and improved moods. Hallelujah! We were all feeling great!

So how would my life have benefited if I'd had the information then that I have now? Why should someone spend years trying to figure this out? This life-changing knowledge that I have found is the whole reason for this book – so that you and anyone else can end the unnecessary suffering. You can feel great, be healthy, and live as vibrantly as you were designed to do.

The secret is now out!

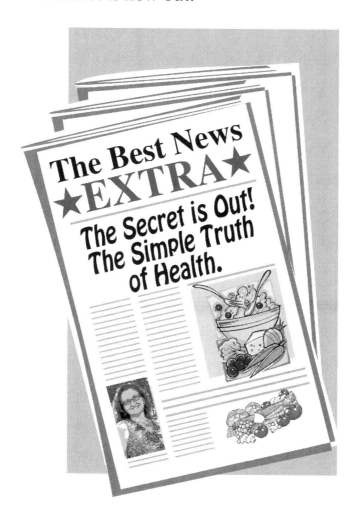

Chapter 1

WHAT'S YOUR 20?

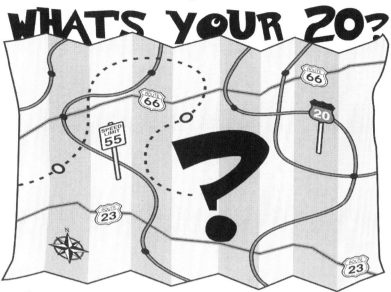

I want to educate drivers and non-drivers alike on the importance of good health. Much of our health comes from the health of our gut. So what is gut health? Gut health is the condition of our digestive system. Whether or not our gut is in top condition determines many

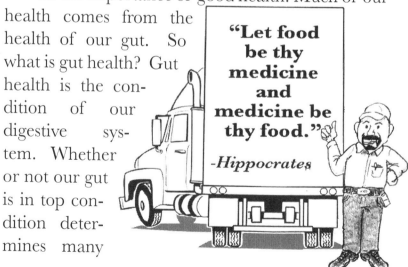

"Let food be thy medicine and medicine be thy food."

-Hippocrates

aspects of how we feel. If our gut is in great shape, we will likely have few health concerns.

After reading this book you will have a better understanding of how to maintain your health on the road. One way to nail down the ideas in this book is to read them over and over. When you read the book once, you will become aware of a certain amount of information and have it to use in your everyday life. When you read it again, you will be at a different place in your thinking and will see other ideas that you didn't catch before. Each and every time you take in the thoughts in this book, you will very likely find something new. This will help you to transition into good habits and remind you of the goals that you have set for yourself.

There is a wide variety of on-the-road situations out there. The long haul drivers range from those with no means of food preparation to those who have a super sleeper with a full kitchen. So, let's determine your food preparation potential. Only you can map out the right direction for you.

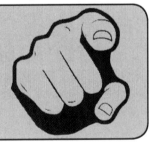

Where there is a will there is a way. Why? Because YOU are worth it!

Ask yourself these questions.

- Is it possible for you to prepare food in the truck?
- Do you have or can you get an inverter?
- Do you need 12 volt appliances?
- What small appliances do you already have?
- What appliances will most fit your lifestyle preferences?
- Are you willing to go that extra mile to do what it takes to be healthy and vibrant?

The No-Cook Plan

Having no means of food preparation does present a challenge to eating quality food, but I am up for the challenge. Are you? This book will provide you with information on the health effects of food prepared with additives versus food prepared naturally. This will teach you to be aware of what to look for and what to leave out in the search for food.

When you are eating out, don't hesitate to ask questions. You never know, there just might be a knowledgeable cook in the back. When you discover what sounds good to you on the menu, think about how it could be altered to cut out the unnecessary additives. Ask what seasonings that they have. If the word seasoning is in it, stay away; it probably has MSG, sugar, and unnecessary additives. Listen for the good, healthy things like pepper, rosemary, garlic, and onion. Just plain single ingredient flavors. These can be added in any quantity and be flavorful and healthy.

Restaurants will almost always use vegetable oil to cook with. Vegetable oil = soybean oil. You will learn about this later. Again, ask if they have any other options of oil to cook with. You never know, they might surprise you and have a good choice available.

Think single foods like green beans and pinto beans. Instead of getting the hash brown casserole, get a baked potato or better yet, a baked sweet potato. Be sure to tell them to make the sweet potato plain. When I have ordered a sweet potato, they put sugar on it. It is great just plain.

Drink good quality water. If possible, bring in your own water. I use the Big Berkey gravity water filtration system at home and love it. Not only will it save you a ton of money, it will cut down on the chemical load in your body. Let's do the math. If you buy water bottles at the truck stop, they will average $1.25 each. At this price, if you only drink 64 ounces per day, you will be spending approximately $1370 per year. If you buy the large packs of bottled water, at the gro-

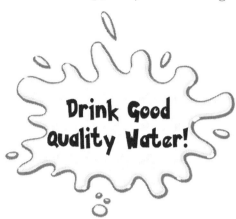

Drink Good Quality Water!

cery store, they average about $.20 each. This will cost you about $200 per year. But if you do some research and find a good quality water filter, such as the Sport Berkey bottle, you will spend about $45 per year. You will know the quality of the water you're drinking, and you'll have the bottle to fill up for free wherever there is a water source. What are your thoughts?

> ***Please note:***
> *Cut down on water thirty minutes or so before a meal. Drinking very little during a meal prevents dilution of stomach acids. Less fluids will help out with digestion.*

Those Of You Who Have A Super Sleeper

Lucky duck! You are very outnumbered and blessed to have such an outfit. With a little ambition and planning, you can make just about anything that you can dream up. CREATE!

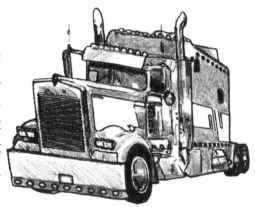

Now For The Majority Of You Drivers

Sure, cleanup is the pits, and it sure would be nice to have some more space. But it is all worth it. Good health and feeling great, inside and out, is priceless. Only you can do it. If you plan right and make wise purchases, you can also save money. Which of the prior questions, at the beginning of this chapter, fit your situation? Let's begin.

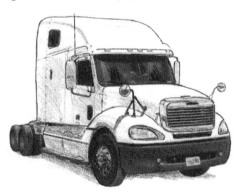

Thoughts to Ponder

1. What are your biggest challenges of being on the road?

2. What concerns do you have about your health?

3. What needs to change about your routine?

4. On a scale of 1 to 10 how committed are you to improving your health?

5. If you are a 10 **GREAT!** What are you waiting for?

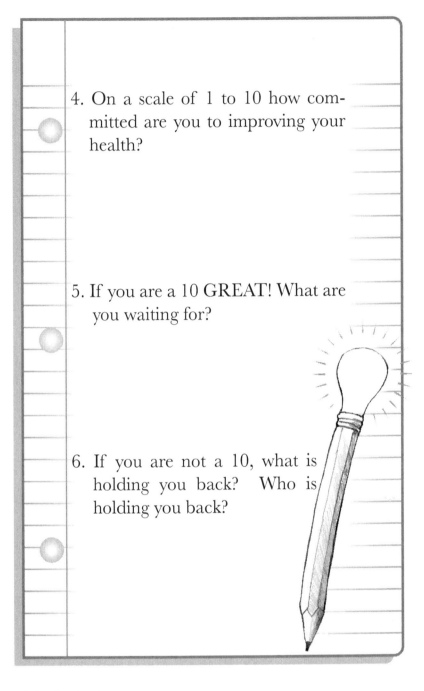

6. If you are not a 10, what is holding you back? Who is holding you back?

7. Make a list of what or who is holding you back.

Deeply examine the answers to these questions. Your answers may be lowering your quality of life or worse they may be shortening your lifespan.

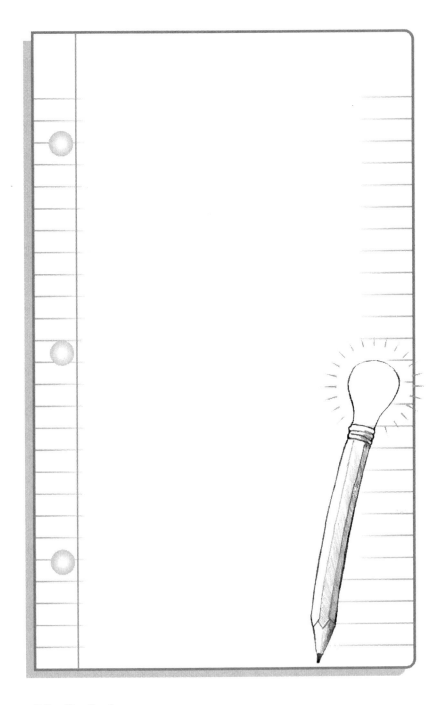

Chapter 2

WHATS IN IT FOR YOU?

Get ready for no gimmicks, no pills, no shakes, and no miracles. I am going to inform you of some plain old simple methods that work by design. They can provide quality of life IF you put them into action. You can do it! Will you?

Have you ever wished you could experience these things daily?

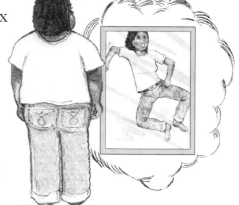

Free from acid reflux
Medication free
Disease reversal
Weight loss
Lubed joints
No C-PAP
Full of energy
Feeling young again
More energy boost
Inner and outer strength
      Better job performance
      Self-worth

This information is very simple. Some of you will conquer it with little or no effort, and others may require more. Either way it is ALL POSSIBLE. It is all possible for you, driver! I have seen this work time and time again and have experienced it myself.

Get off the road to dis - ease and get ready for the ride of your life!

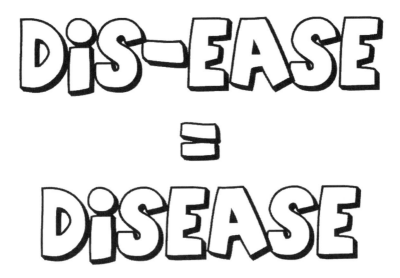

Thoughts to Ponder

1. How do you feel about feeling good?

2. What things could you do if you had spring in your step again?

3. How would your life change if the aches and pains were not there?

4. What are some of the best things about feeling vibrant and healthy?

5. What would be better in your life if medicine were out of the picture?

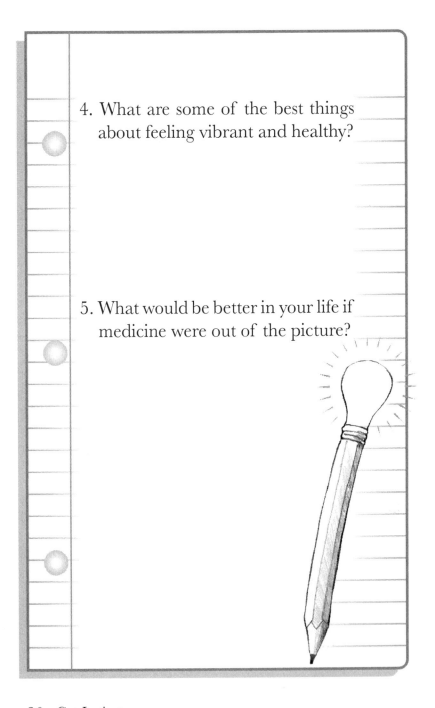

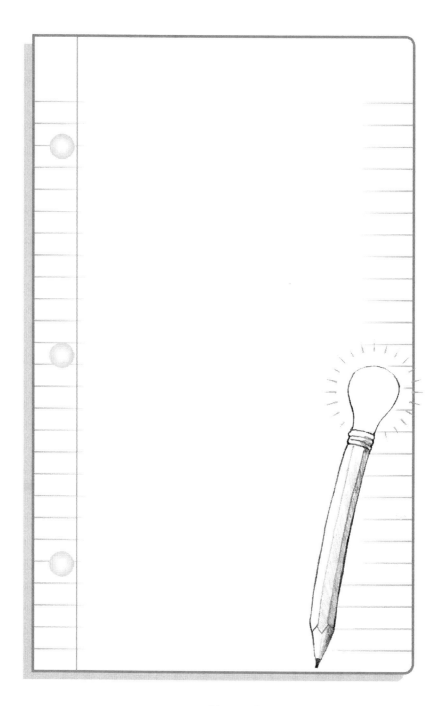

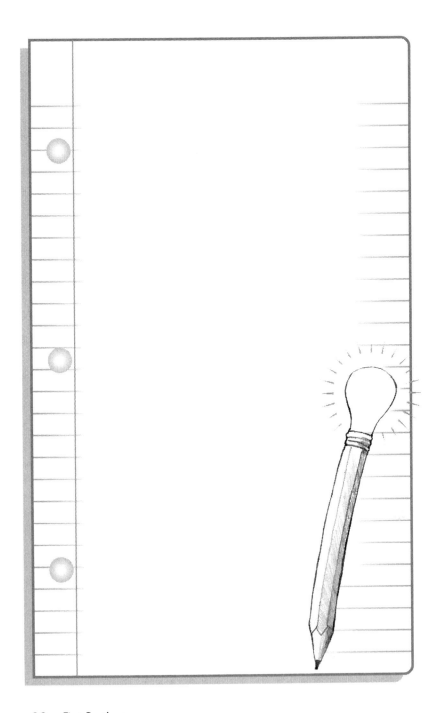

Chapter 3

YOU ARE IN THE DRIVER'S SEAT!

Drivers, I feel as if I would be doing you an injustice if I didn't go into the subject of choices before we jump into the many gears of gut health.

Knowing information sometimes just isn't enough to create an awareness for the need of an overall change in the improving of our health. Many times we know the information, but we don't do what we know is best. Are you in control of what happens in your life, or do external situations control you? Let me give you an example.

There are two individual drivers going down the interstate, and both are heading home. Traffic comes to a standstill with no information of the problem or the time frame of clearing. One of the guys is calling home to inform his family of the change. He is using this time to speak with them, asking about their day, making different plans, and so on. Hanging up, after much visiting on the phone, he then starts to sing along with the radio and begins thinking of the things that he needs to do when he gets home.

The other guy starts getting frustrated. He calls home in anger to tell his family why he will be late. Then he starts banging on the steering wheel and yelling profane things. He decides to get out of his truck to see if he can tell what's going on while still ranting. Someone tells him to settle down, and that infuriates him even more.

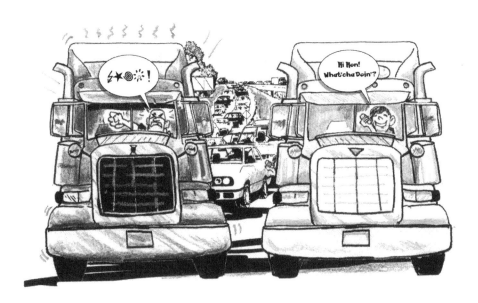

Which person's situation will get them out of the traffic jam faster? These types of choices may not seem important at the time but are very important to every aspect of our lives. The way we see things and react to them makes all the difference in the world, sometimes life changing differences. Which one of these two situations best describes you? Do you let circumstances control you, or are you in control of how you respond to circumstances around you?

In the case of our health, these choices can determine whether we have a high or low quality of life. If we don't have quality of life, what good is life? Why should we go through life with physical or emotional pain that can be prevented? It is impossible for someone else to make an inner change for you. You are going to choose to apply this information for your highest good, or you are going to take it in and do nothing about it.

Exercise your mental muscle. Think of how you want to be and make it happen.

Will this book fire up your creative engine to do something about the quality of your life? Will it be such an awakening that you are going to have the "no matter what" attitude that will instantly kick in? Can you see your potential? Take a moment and close your eyes. Picture yourself free from all aches, pains, health concerns, emotional issues, or any negative state of being. See yourself happy, healthy, and feeling young again. Well, is it worth it? Is a change in thought and behavior worth that wonderful, healthy, vibrant you?

Some of us get a hold of great information and get pumped up about it, buy the product, and there it sits one year later. Why is it that we want to do something to change our lives, but we don't do it? Who we are is a gathering of habits, practices, beliefs, attitudes, and expectations that may or may not be ours. WHAT? Explain that one to me again. Yes, who we are is a mix of beliefs that our parents, grandparents, aunts, uncles, TV, radio, or any other external force has put ideas into our minds. As children, we didn't have a choice of what information went into our minds. We were like sponges and accepted all ideas suggested to us or shown to us by example. As we get older we have a choice of what we can keep or kick out of our minds. Many times we are in a situation that we realize is not how we want it to be, but we are comfortable with it. It seems that it is easier for us to stay in a situation that we realize is not good for us, than it is to get out of that comfort zone and change our situation. Let's take a big rig for example, someone programmed it to run a certain way. It has no choice but to run exactly as it was programmed. We, on the other hand, do have a choice. We can change that programming if we want to badly enough.

Let's look at where you are now and look at where you want to be. Get a sheet of paper. At the top of the page write down your present situation. At the bottom, write where and who you want to be. Then draw a straight line from your present situation to your goal. Write on that line what has to be done to get from point A to

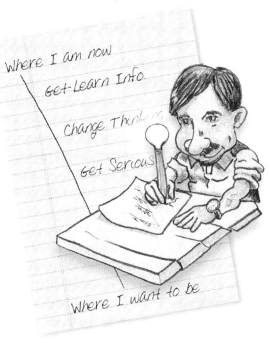

point B, just as you map out the run you have been given. The closer you stay to that line the faster you are going to get there. If you stick to the route that you have laid out, you will get there in fewer miles and make good time. Make a plan so that you can stay on track. Keep your eye on the goal. No right or left turns, and definitely no U turns.

Think of this. Check your calendar and your checkbook. These two places will show you where you have placed your priorities and decisions in the past. Now that you 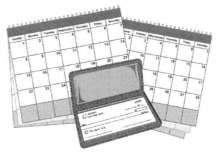 have this realization, commit to it, and let's see you soar. Let's see how different that calendar and check- book look this time next year.

Remember you are truly the only thing that you can control. Don't let something else, like bad hab- its or someone else's ideas control you. By the end of this book you will have plenty of information on board to direct your path down the road to your success in health.

Thoughts to Ponder

1. Make a list of past choices that you want to change. What are the top three?

2. How can choosing to react positively to circumstances affect the following:

   Your self worth?

Your relationships?

Your productivity?

Your job?

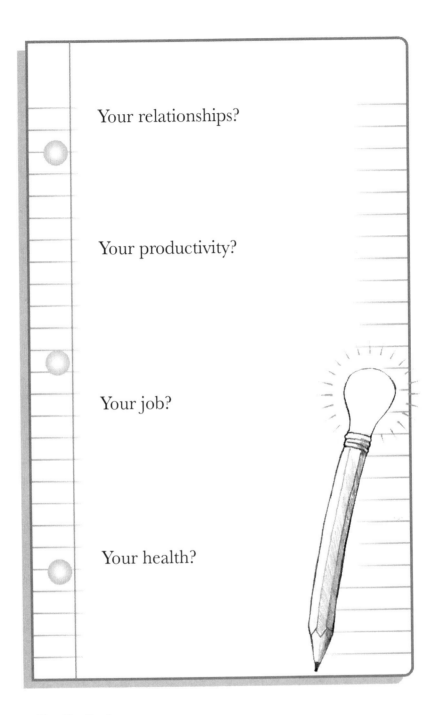

Your health?

3. What can you do about it?

4. Who can help you?

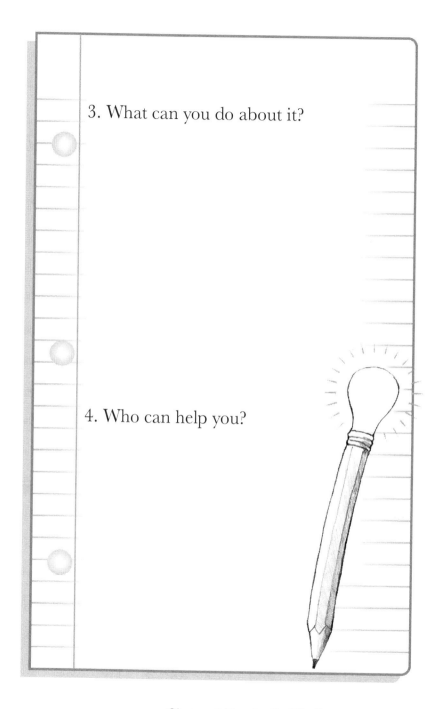

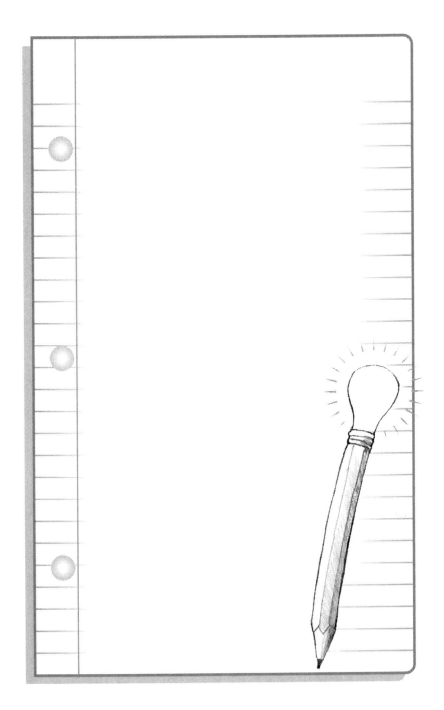

Chapter 4

WHY SHOULD I LOVE MY GUTS?

Our digestive system starts at our lips and ends when we have a bowel movement. When I speak of guts I am talking about the inner part of our intestine. In other words, our gut is the part of our intestines that our food moves through.

Lots of people don't realize the enormous role and importance that our gut plays in health and wellness. It all starts in our mouths by using saliva and chewing to give the digestive process a kick start. How we chew our food and how long we chew it is very important. We should chew our food for however long it takes to make it into a complete mush before swallowing. This is an important yet simple step that many hurry through before the task is complete.

When the food reaches the stomach, a new process takes place. This time it is more like a chemical reaction. The stomach produces enzymes and HCl. YEP, hydrochloric acid. Some of you tanker drivers may have had to haul this. When the chewed food comes in contact with HCl, the stomach churns it all around and breaks it down into tiny particles, turning it into a milkshake consistency. This process is very important.

The next destination is the small intestine. This is where things get really interesting. Here is where most of the nutrients are absorbed. Until we absorb these nutrients, they are of absolutely no benefit. Common sense tells us that no nutrients or fuel = no health. Can your truck run without fuel? Boy, don't we wish. . . .

So, if you eat high-nutrient foods, will you be healthy? Well, yes and no. It all depends on what shape your gut is in. Have you given it what it needs and fed it the food that it was designed to get in order for it to work correctly? If it is not in tip top shape, there is a good chance that you are not absorbing the nutrients that you are eating and getting the benefit of good health. Let's find out what can happen to our gut and what causes it to be unhealthy.

Within our digestive tract exists a living ecosystem. Ideally, the good guys should largely outnumber the bad; however, many times this is not the case. So, what happens when we eat these added and altered ingredients? We throw off the balance of our gut's bacteria. We look into this subject in the chapter *"The Mechanics Of It."*

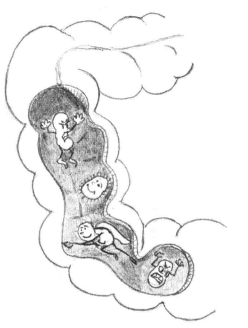

The word *food* is one that we take for granted. We tend to think that anything we eat can be categorized as *food*. But the word *food* has a specific definition. For example, a person could eat a piece of gum, but that doesn't mean that gum is *food*. The free dictionary defines *food* as material, usually of plant or animal origin, that contains or consists of essential body nutrients, such as carbohydrates, fats, proteins, vitamins, or minerals, and is ingested and assimilated by an organism to produce energy, stimulate growth, and maintain life.[1] Do fast food and processed food fit this definition?

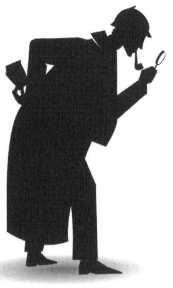

Be Your Own Private Investigator

Let's take a look at what some of us eat. Our current food supply is a far cry from how we were designed to eat. As recently as fifty years ago, it was a treat to get something processed or not homemade. Now it is a treat not to get processed food and to get something homemade. Keep in mind the definition of homemade has also drastically changed over the years. Nowadays the majority of what we eat has some or all of these ingredients: (If you eat processed foods it is near 100%.)

Corn	Preservatives
Soy	Nitrates and nitrites
Wheat	Artificial color
Sugar	MSG
Artificial flavors	Excess amounts of sodium
Artificial sweeteners	

Well, I can maybe see why artificial sweeteners, artificial colors, artificial flavors, preservatives, nitrates, nitrites, and MSG might be bad, but how are the others bad? Aren't they "natural?"

I highly encourage you to begin a quest to search the Internet for information on the horrible health effects of the unnatural ingredients that you may be eating.

—m— Corn —m—

Let's start with corn. Natural, right? It should be, shouldn't it? According to the USDA, over 89% of corn grown in the U.S. is a GMO (genetically modified organism).[2]

*Challenge:

Search "health effects of GMO corn" on the Internet.

(Hint: Dr. Mercola's site has some very eye-opening information on GMO.)

Here is a list of some health effects that the website *Responsible Technology* shares.

Allergies

Allergic reactions

Liver problems

Reproductive problems

Infant mortality

Sterility

(This information is not only for ladies.)

Death

There are many more than this, but you get the picture.

—⟋⟍— **Soy** —⟋⟍—

According to the USDA, 94% of soy is a GMO (genetically modified organism).[3] Have you read the ingredients of the food that you are eating lately?

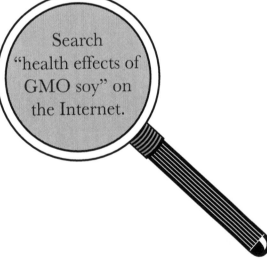

Search "health effects of GMO soy" on the Internet.

*Challenge:

What are genetically modified organisms? They are seeds that have been genetically altered to carry on a certain behavior. GMO corn and soy, for instance, are altered so that they are still be able to thrive even after being sprayed with a chemical that kills all other nearby vegetation, like weeds. This chemical alone is very bad for our health. These seeds have also been changed genetically to have their own capabilities to resist fungi, viruses, bacteria, diseases, and insects. If we eat this, is it causing the same things to happen in our gut? Since we have an abundance of beneficial bacteria, viruses, and fungi in our gut, this altered food can kill off these microbes that are designed to be in our digestive system. I don't want to be eating these chemicals. Do you?

—ᵔ— Meat —ᵔ—

What about the animals that eat GMO's? Unless naturally raised, these animals are not only subjected to cruel treatment, they are fed almost completely GMO products. They have such mass production and horrible conditions that their digestive systems can't work properly, thus causing reason to need antibiotics and other medications. As you will see in the recipes, I am for animal products in moderation if that is your choice, but only animal products that have been raised, fed, and treated in a way that they were designed to be.

For instance, I see in the stores all the time, "all natural vegetarian-fed chicken." It can't be all natural, because chickens are not vegetarians. We've all heard this, "corn-fed beef." Think back to the old ranching days, cows grazed on grass, not corn, especially not GMO corn.

Although good choices are out there to find, they are not as readily available as they should be. As a matter of fact, all food should be responsibly raised and we should not have to look farther than our local store. The more demand for a high quality of food, the more available it will become. Search out where to find the best sources. They are there; you just don't know it. Please check out all the information on this yourself and be VERY picky about the meat that you eat.

⚊ᔕᔕ Dairy ᔕᔕ⚊

Dairy comes from animals fed the same way as described in the "Meat" section. The cows are fed GMOs and are given substances that are designed to make them produce many times more gallons of milk than they are designed to produce. This creates

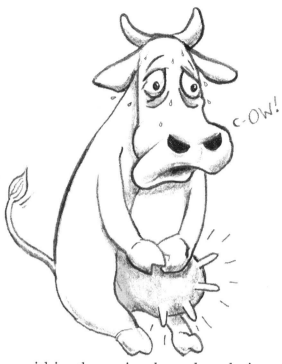

problems within the animal, and a chain reaction occurs which causes it to need more substances such as antibiotics to overcome the other problems associated with the first issue, and a vicious cycle begins.

A huge percentage of the population has an intolerance to milk. It is my thinking that we are designed to be weaned off our mother's milk by a couple of years old. All milk-producing animals have a weaning period. A cow's milk is designed to fortify an 85 pound infant into a 250 to 270 pound calf at about 8 months old. Then add the fact that they have very often been given milk that has been altered. This is not natural nor healthy and contributes to the irritation of our guts. But if you choose to eat it, keep in mind that eating only organic is very important.

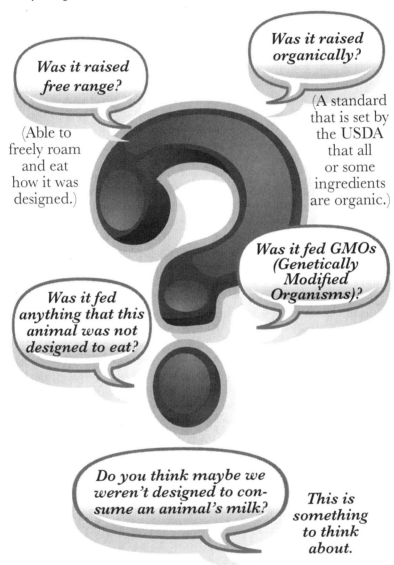

Was it raised free range?

(Able to freely roam and eat how it was designed.)

Was it raised organically?

(A standard that is set by the USDA that all or some ingredients are organic.)

Was it fed anything that this animal was not designed to eat?

Was it fed GMOs (Genetically Modified Organisms)?

Do you think maybe we weren't designed to consume an animal's milk?

This is something to think about.

Grains

Grains in their natural form can be healthy. <u>IF</u> the grains we eat were grown and processed properly, and <u>IF</u> our digestive systems were in tip-top shape, we should not have issues when eating grains. The problem is that most of our digestive systems are compromised. A gut that is not in good shape will usually have a very hard time digesting grains. So in order to get the gut in shape we have to give it a break from this disturbance. If you are serious about getting your gut back in shape the grains will have to go, for now.

Here is a list of grains to look for on the label of ingredients:

- •Barley
- •Bulgur wheat
- •Corn
- •Durum wheat
- •Fonio
- •Kamut
- •Millet
- •Oats
- •Popcorn
- •Rice
- •Rye
- •Semolina wheat
- •Sorghum
- •Spelt
- •Teff
- •Triticale
- •Wheat
- •Wild rice

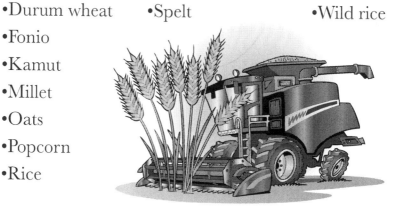

—ₘ— Wheat —ₘ—

☺Good news – most wheat is not a GMO.

☹Bad news – Because of the condition that most of us have within our guts, some foods can irritate and trigger allergic responses more than others. Wheat is one of these triggers. Wheat is also, in most cases very contaminated with many chemicals to keep it pest, weed, and disease free. This alone can be detrimental to our health.

Wheat and other grains also contain gluten. According to some researchers, none of us can digest gluten. If left undigested, the potential is there to cause problems. Wheat also has a high glycemic index. Those of you with diabetes sure know what this means. Not only does this cause a problem in people with diabetes, it also contributes to deep visceral fat (belly fat) and atherosclerotic plaque (a plaque build up inside your arteries), which can trigger heart disease and stroke.

What about fiber? Most of the wheat eaten in this country is so processed that there is hardly any fiber left. Even if you choose whole wheat bread, the main ingredient is usually a very processed flour. Eating a diet consisting of lots of fruits and vegetables can provide all the fiber that you'll ever need.

Most of us realize that too much sugar is bad for us. If not, the artificial sugars wouldn't be so popular. We need some natural sugars to be healthy, but it needs to be the right kind of sugar in the correct amounts. If we never added sugar to anything and ate a good variety of natural foods, we would have a sufficient amount sugar for health. White 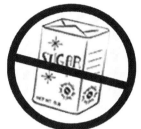 sugar has no vitamins, minerals, or nutrients at all. It is just empty calories. Corn syrup, from genetically modified corn, has no nutrients and is said to be even more harmful than cane sugar. And don't forget about sugar beets. They are also GMO and account for a large portion of the added sugar in our foods. Yes, some sugars are more harmful than others, but the bottom line is that an excess of any sugars will create negative health effects.

According to the Mayo Clinic,[4] added sugar sets the stage for potential health problems, such as:

Weight Gain

Increased Triglycerides

Poor Nutrition

Tooth Decay

Do you know someone affected by any of these?

And according to Authoritynutrition.com,[5] added sugar can also do the following:

•Overload your liver

•Cause insulin resistance, raising the risk of type 2 diabetes

•Cause cancer

•Affect hormones

•Cause addiction

•Raise cholesterol

•Cause heart disease

I did some research on the Internet to find out how much sugar the average person consumes, and I got answers that ranged from about 130 pounds to 170 pounds per year. Whichever one is right is a ridiculous amount to consume.

One of the many ways that sugar is harmful to the gut is that it feeds the bad bacteria. This creates an overgrowth of the bad vs. the good.

—ᴧᴧ— Artificial Sweeteners —ᴧᴧ—

Again, Dr. Mercola has some good information on artificial sweeteners. Here is a list from his site of the negative effects of **aspartame**.[6]

Headaches/migraines
Dizziness
Muscle spasms
Irritability
Heart palpitations
Tinnitus (Ringing in the ears)
Weight gain
Tachycardia
Breathing difficulties
Vertigo
Seizures
Nausea

Numbness
Rashes
Depression
Fatigue
Insomnia
Vision problems
Hearing loss
Anxiety attacks
Slurred speech
Memory loss
Joint pain
Loss of taste

Solve this mystery:

How do they make aspartame?

You will be totally grossed out!

The website also listed some symptoms of Splenda. These include the following:

Gastrointestinal problems
Seizures, dizziness, and migraines
Blurred vision
Allergic reactions
Blood sugar increases and weight gain

The featured review also concluded that sucralose destroys gut bacteria.[7]

Preservatives, Artificial Colors, Nitrates, And Nitrites

Also from mercola.com some information on preservatives, artificial colors, nitrates and nitrites:

BHT . . .
neurological problems, behavioral issues, hormonal issues, metabolic dysfunction, and cancer.

TBHQ . . .
Nausea and vomiting, tinnitus, delirium, sense of suffocation, liver toxicity, reproductive mutations.

Sodium Nitrite and Nitrate . . .
colorectal, stomach, and pancreatic cancers.

Azodicarbonamide . . .

cancer, asthma, allergies

Artificial Colors . . .

nine of the food dyes currently approved for use in the US are linked to health issues ranging from cancer to hyperactivity and allergy-like reactions.[8]

—~~—MSG —~~—

What is it? Why do they use it?

MSG, or monosodium glutamate, is a neurotoxin and an excitotoxin. What does this mean?

A neurotoxin is a substance that toxifies or inhibits the function of a neuron. A neuron is simply a nerve cell. These poisons can range from severely damaging the cell so that is doesn't function at all, to interfering with the way it works.

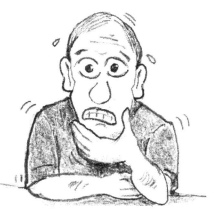

MSG is a substance with many names. If you look on the label for MSG, you might not see it in the ingredients. This does not indicate an absence of it.

According to truthinlabeling.org, this list of ingredients will always contain processed free glutamic acid, MSG[9]

Glutamic acid (E 620)2

Glutamate (E 620)

Monosodium glutamate (E 621)

Monopotassium glutamate (E 622)

Calcium glutamate (E 623)

Monoammonium glutamate (E 624)

Magnesium glutamate (E 625)

Natrium glutamate

Anything "hydrolyzed"

Any "hydrolyzed protein"

Calcium caseinate, Sodium caseinate

Anything "enzyme modified"

Anything containing "enzymes"

Anything "fermented"

Anything containing "protease"

Vetsin

Ajinomoto

Umami

Yeast extract, Torula yeast

Yeast food, Yeast nutrient

Autolyzed yeast

Gelatin

Textured protein

Whey protein

Whey protein concentrate

Whey protein isolate

Soy protein

Soy protein concentrate

Soy protein isolate

Anything "protein"

Anything "protein fortified"

Soy sauce

Soy sauce extract

In addition, some other neurotoxins include:

Aspartame (also known as Equal, Amino Sweet, NutraSweet, Spoonful)

Sucralose (also known as Splenda)

Fluoride (sodium fluoride)

An excitotoxin is a substance that excites our neurons. In reality it excites our taste buds to make bland food taste wonderful, therefore contributing to cravings and overeating.

Many other adverse effects have also been linked to regular consumption of MSG, including the following:

Obesity

Eye damage

Headaches

Fatigue and disorientation

Depression

According to the Mayo Clinic, even the FDA admits that "short-term reactions" known as MSG Symptom Complex can occur in certain groups of people, namely those who have eaten "large doses" of MSG or those who have asthma.[10] According to the FDA, MSG Symptom Complex can involve symptoms such as:

Numbness

Burning sensation

Tingling

Facial pressure or tightness

Chest pain or difficulty breathing

Headache

Nausea

Rapid heartbeat

Drowsiness

Weakness

Now that we have touched on what can happen to our gut and what causes it to be unhealthy, and we have found out a little bit about some of the additives in processed food, look back at the definition of the word *food*. Do any of these items fall under the category of *food*?

You decide.

Endnotes

1 http://www.thefreedictionary.com/food

2 United States Department of Agriculture. (2015 July 9). "Adoption of Genetically Engineered Crops in the U.S." http://www.ers.usda.gov/data-products/adoption-of-genetically-engineered-crops-in-the-us/recent-trends-in-ge-adoption.aspx

3 Ibid.

4 Mayo Clinic Staff (2016 January. 24) Added sugars: Don't get sabotaged by sweeteners http://www.mayoclinic.org/healthy-lifestyle/nutrition-and-healthy-eating/in-depth/added-sugar/art-20045328

5 Gunnars, Kris (2013 September) "10 Disturbing Reasons Why Sugar is Bad For You." http://authoritynutrition.com/10-disturbing-reasons-why-sugar-is-bad/

6 (2011 November 6) "Aspartame: By Far the Most Dangerous Substance Added to Most Foods Today." http://articles.mercola.com/sites/articles/archive/2011/11/06/aspartame-most-dangerous-subsance-added-to-food.aspx

7 Mercola, Joseph. (2009 February 10). "New Study of Splenda (Sucratose) Reveals Shocking Information About Potential Harmful Effects" http://articles.mercola.com/sites/articles/archives/2009/02/10/news-study-of-splenda-rveals-shocking-information-about-potential-harmful-effects.aspx

8 Mercola, Joseph. (2015 March 18). "The Eight Most Damaging Ingredients to Watch for on Food Labels." http://articles.mercola.com/sites/articles/archives/2015/03/18/8-worst-processed-food-ingredients.aspx

9 Truth in Labeling Campaign. (2014 March). "Names of ingredients that contain processed free glutanic acid (MSG)." http://www.truthinlabeling.org/hiddensources.html

10 Zeratsky, Katherine. (2015 March 13). "Nutrition and Healthy Eating." http://www.mayoclinic.org/healthy-lifestyle/nutrition-and-healthy-eating/expert-answers/monosodium-glutamate/faq-20058196

Thoughts to Ponder

1. What did you discover about GMO?

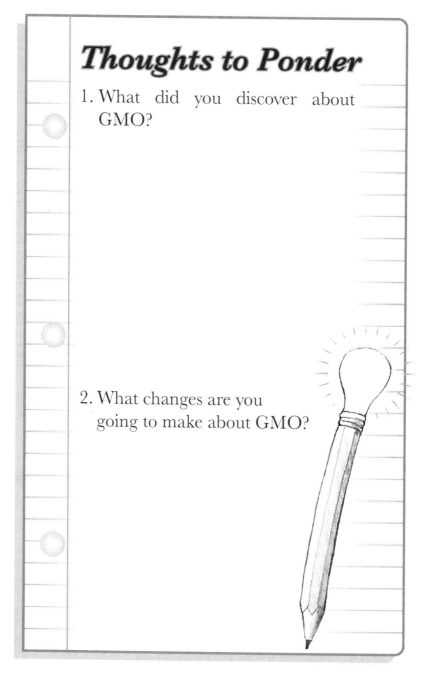

2. What changes are you going to make about GMO?

3. What did you discover about food additives?

4. How have additives impacted your health?

5. How does this make you feel?

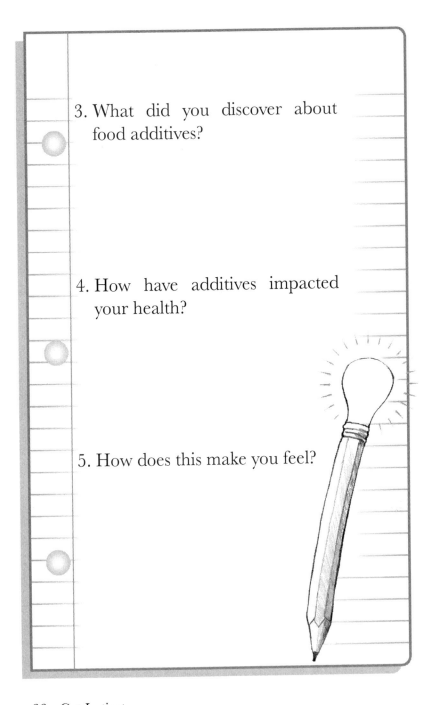

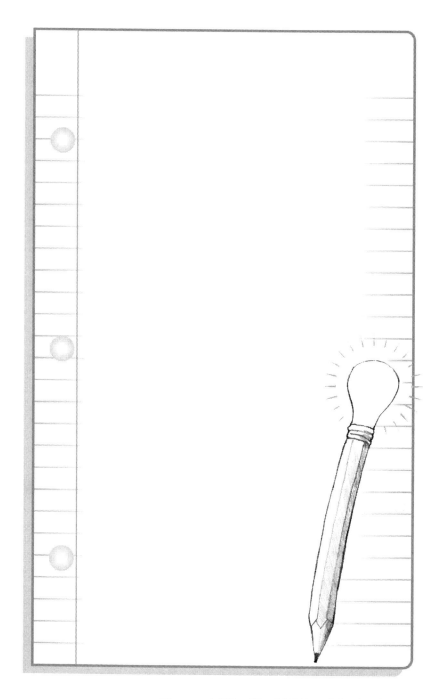

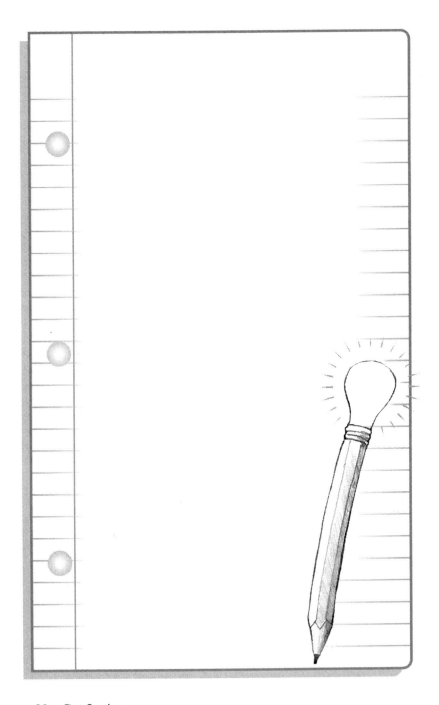

Chapter 5

The Mechanics of It!

So now that you know why you should love your gut, here is how it works. What role does your gut play in your health or lack thereof?

Not only does your gut digest food and absorb nutrients and water, it also produces vital nutrients that you need. Some of these nutrients are cultivated by the organisms living there.

Let's look into absorbing nutrients. As mentioned earlier, when food gets into the small intestine, it is the consistency of a milkshake, broken down into tiny particles that are then absorbed through the walls of the small intestine. I want you to picture this. Think of a soaker hose. You know; you can get them in the garden center at any hardware store. They lay in your flower beds to slowly water the ground. The water seeps through tiny holes that you cannot see. This is how our small intestines are designed to work. Many of us, however, have small intestines that have been abused by processed foods, stress, and medications, which cause the holes in your small intestine to enlarge.

Instead of the tiny nutrients in this slush being able to seep through tiny holes, the holes have become larger, like a net instead of a soaker hose, letting larger particles through. This is a big problem and is called leaky gut syndrome. One of the many issues that may stem from leaky gut is allergies. When the larger particles escape our gut lining, our immune system tags them as invaders. When these larger particles invade, our inner army comes to the rescue and is ready to fight, sometimes worsening each time to a point of an anaphylactic reaction, which can cause death.

Commonly, the immune system flips on the mucus switch in order to wash the invader away. This may happen in our gut, sinuses, lungs, or somewhere in between. This battle in the immune system can cause itching, burning, watering, reddening, welts, constriction, swelling, fever, rashes, or a number of other different symptoms that many of us have experienced. Have you experienced any of these? It can also turn on inflammation wherever it wants, usually in your weakest areas. Joints and organs are common places for inflammation to occur. Allergic reactions very often occur on our skin, which is our biggest organ, causing eczema, psoriasis, dry skin, flaky skin, and breakouts. As you can see, when our bodies are in constant turmoil, it's no wonder that we don't feel well.

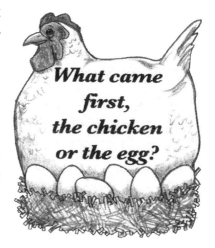

What came first, the chicken or the egg?

—∿— **Stress** —∿—

Are you stressed because your gut is compromised or is your gut compromised because you are stressed? Both ways, stress has a huge impact on all functions of our body and the way that we feel. Have you been in a stressful situation and felt butterflies, heartburn, indigestion, or gas?

This is no coincidence. All of our bodily functions are connected, especially our brain and gut. Even people who eat right can suffer from digestive issues caused by stress.

Have you ever heard about fight or flight? This is where our body kicks in the adrenaline. We can run faster and farther than we ever thought we could, and we can pick up objects heavier than we could imagine. When we are in this state of being, all of our bodily systems put total emphasis on the area of concern. This means, if we are running from a bear, our body is not worried about that stuffy nose that we might have. It is putting all efforts into our legs to run as fast and as long as we can to get away. When this is happening, that stuffy nose is not very important any more, and there is no energy being given to it. Many people live daily in a state of fight or flight. Living this way takes all the energy that we need to maintain and heal our bodies and puts it into other areas that are sending false alarms.

This stress can actually change the chemicals and the makeup of our gut. Remember the living eco-system in our gut? Stress can alter this and get it out of balance. Stress-induced leaky gut is the change in the permeability of our small and large intestine from allowing small particles to pass through to letting larger particles pass (turning that soaker hose that we talked about earlier into a net). Leaky gut is the culprit of many different types of diseases. This means stress can contribute to, or actually cause, many of the digestive issues that occur today.

Take Charge!

First you must become aware of the stress that is within you. There are many ways to do this. If you are that determined go-getter type, you can do 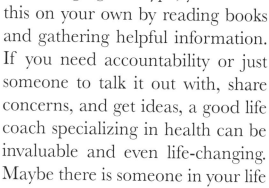 this on your own by reading books and gathering helpful information. If you need accountability or just someone to talk it out with, share concerns, and get ideas, a good life coach specializing in health can be invaluable and even life-changing. Maybe there is someone in your life who is dedicated to your highest good, like a friend or family member, that will work with you. Give yourself permission to receive comfort and guidance from others, and be sure to choose wisely.

Many people have high levels of chronic stress and don't even realize it.

Examine yourself, how do you react to outside situations? Do certain things trigger anger, frustration, or any type of emotional outburst? Even when there are no occurrences, do you still feel uptight, tense, or like something is wrong?

Be your own personal private investigator, not only in examining your emotions, but also in inspecting the food that you eat. Write down what you have discovered about your stress levels and what the triggers are. Make a plan of what to do when the triggers occur, so that when they happen, you'll know how to respond.

Also, make a commitment to take the time to meditate. There are many good places on YouTube that can help you discover how to meditate. You can do this when you're on a driving break by simply closing your eyes and thinking about happy things and goals. Sometimes things need to be dealt with immediately. It's ok to make a quick stop to regroup. Go in your mind to a place of peace and tranquility, like somewhere tropical, or think of a memorable happy moment in your past that brings a smile to your face.

As you are driving down the road, instead of thinking of negative things and worrying, reflect on happy thoughts, dreams, and ideas. Visualize the person you want to be. Search your thoughts for what things you need to do in order to be this new, improved you. Who knows, this thinking might spur an invention or idea that changes the way that we live today. Also, listening to music or books that have positive meaning is an awesome way to start changing your thought process right now.

Water, why is it important?

How and where does our gut absorb water? Most of us don't drink enough water. A good way to figure out about how much water that we need is to divide your weight in half and drink that many ounces. For example, if you weigh 150 pounds you would want to make a goal of drinking 75 ounces per day.

Quality water is very important. The water that comes out of the tap is not quality water. The best choice is to find a good source of spring water. Be forewarned. This is not always an easy task. If quality spring water is not easily available, be sure to get highly filtered water. This should be pretty easy to come by at large stores. Just try to read the origination and procedures to filter it, or get your own filter.

Drinking a lot of water all at once is good for flushing the kidneys. This is very important to know if you have a tendency of getting UTIs (urinary tract infection). But drinking water all throughout the day, especially an hour or so before meals, is typically the best method. Drinking water throughout the day ensures a steady flow of water to hydrate our bodies. However, drinking during meals dilutes the acids in our stomach which causes our food not to digest properly.

—ᴡ— **Ideas** —ᴡ—

Keep water with you at all times, so it is always convenient.

Get in a routine for drinking water. Set an alarm for every thirty minutes to an hour to drink eight ounces. Be sure to skip the drink before eating. There are also apps that you can download that will help you keep track of your water intake.

Realize how much money you will save by keeping hydrated and only drinking water and not chemical and sugar-laden drinks.

This alone will help you lose weight. Adding freshly squeezed lemon helps to flush toxins and adds nutrients. Store bought flavored water or flavored water packets do NOT count.

Make your good choices as easy as possible to get to. The more convenient it is to access, the more likely you are to grab it instead of something else unhealthy. Being hydrated also makes you feel good. Some symptoms of dehydration are dry mouth, sleepiness, dry skin, constipation, headache, dizziness, irritability, and decreased urination. If you are drinking plenty of water all day and still feel thirsty, see your doctor.

So here is the reason water is so important for our gut. The colon (large intestine) absorbs about 80% of the water that we put into our bodies. The longer the stool stays in the colon the more water it absorbs. If it stays too long, the stool will become dry and you will become constipated. Drinking enough water not only helps our kidneys function properly, but it also ensures the proper functioning of our colon.

—₩— Our Inner Ecosystem —₩—

What about those critters living inside of us that I mentioned before? For those of you who love interesting facts like I do, here's one for you. According to smithsonianmag.org, our bodies are made up of 37.2 trillion cells.[1] What is even more interesting is, the common thought that we have ten times that number of microorganisms that live within us and most of them are in our gut. Here is what this number looks like - 37,200,000,000,000,000. But according to National Geographic that number may have been wrong. They are thinking that it is closer to an equal amount of our human cells to microorganisms within us.[2]

If we killed off all of these little critters, we would die. In one form or another they all have jobs. Some produce vitamins such as, K, B1, B2, B6, B12, and biotin, and some are there just to help each other out. It's like having a small living factory inside us. These little guys populate a certain ratio of good to bad in order to keep us healthy. When this ratio gets out of balance, and the bad bacteria take over, there will be problems.

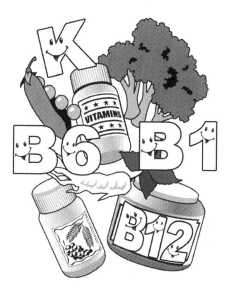

One of the most common issues when this happens is an overgrowth of candida. Candida, sometimes called yeast, is a persistent fungus that is very hard to correct. It loves to eat sugar and starches and is very detrimental to our health. When there is an overgrowth, it seems like it takes control of us. When it's not happy it is sure to let us know about it. The website www.yeastconnection.com gives us a list of some of these problems:

Lack of Focus   Rectal or Vaginal Discomfort
Irritability   Lack of Sexual Feelings
Depressed   Numb
Moody   Dizzy
Crave Sugar   Insomnia[3]
Sleepy

Another website, www.thecandidadiet.com has a more inclusive list of problems associated with a buildup of candida.[4] They include:

Food cravings   Acid reflux
Bloating   Gas
Nausea   Diarrhea
Constipation   Stomach cramps
Night sweats   Psoriasis
Eczema   Dermatitis
Athlete's foot   Body odor
Bad breath   Flu-like symptoms
Hay fever symptoms   Sinusitis
Asthma   Sinus congestion
Chronic post-nasal drip Cysts
Fungal rash   Indigestion
Mucus in stool   Swollen lower lip

Fungal infections of the nails & skin
Thrush (white coating on tongue)
Metallic taste in mouth

Burping after meals
Hemorrhoids
Itching anus
Hives
Canker sores
Bleeding gums
Persistent cough
Sore throat
Eye pain
Itchy eyes
Sensitivity to light
Ear infections
Canker sores

Bleeding gums
Cracked tongue
Persistent cough
Mucus in throat
Sore throat
Sinus congestion
Blurred vision
Bags under eyes
Ringing in the ears
Recurring yeast infections
Inability to lose weight
Frequent colds and flu
Hay fever symptoms

Recurring UTI's (urinary tract infections)
Cystitis (inflammation of the bladder)
PMS & menstrual irregularities
Allergies
Sensitivities to food, fragrances, and chemicals
Headaches
Heart palpitations
Chronic body pain and/or joint pain
Muscle aches and stiffness
Acne

In addition, candida produces waste, and this can also produce its own set of problems. When we do begin to get a hold on the candida overgrowth, and the good bacteria starts to multiply, a die off occurs. This can also cause a list of issues.

Now is a good time to mention detoxing. As we start the process of improving our gut, there can be times when we feel some side effects that are not so pleasant. So, if you are doing all the right things and for some reason are not feeling well, this could be the culprit. Don't get discouraged. Even though our bodies are harmed by unnatural things that we eat, they can become used to them being around. When you stop eating the things that are harmful, our bodies can go through a detox to help get rid of the unwanted substance.

Now let's switch gears to another amazing task that our gut accomplishes. When it's in a healthy state, our gut produces much needed chemicals called neurotransmitters - about forty different ones - one of them being serotonin. Ninety percent of this particular neurotransmitter originates in the gut and is responsible for many important roles in our body. It helps the bowels to function properly, and it lets us know when we have had enough to eat. Serotonin also plays an important role in our moods, whether we feel well or not, and whether or not we

Happy Gut = Happy Person

experience anxiety. It works with our blood to form clots. A lack of it can lead to an increase in osteoporosis. It can add to depression and behavioral disorders, and it helps in regulating sleep. Overall, it helps to regulate our neurons in order to give us a feeling of well-being.

If your serotonin levels are too low or too high, ask the question why? Why are these neurotransmitters off balance?

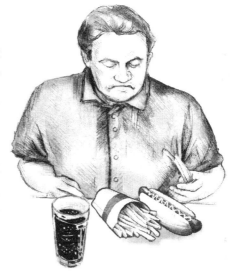

When our gut is not working properly, how can we expect it to follow through with the functions that it was designed to do? Healing the gut is not only about feeling better health-wise, it is also about feeling better emotionally. Everything we eat has a consequence. This consequence can be one of benefit to us, or it can be one of destruction.

Some ideas that are necessary to boost gut improvement, other than eating the right foods, are taking probiotics and eating foods that have these probiotic microorganisms in them. We need these organisms in our gut to sustain the flora that our gut is designed to have. I have chosen to keep about three different brands of probiotics available to use for my family. The reason for this is that each and every brand is going to have some differences in their strains of organisms. These differences will add more variety of the good guys to the gut. Having more variety helps to keep the bad guys under control. There are many different brands and qualities of probiotics available. I would not rely on drug stores or department stores for quality probiotic products. Find a local health food store or a larger health food chain. These places should be able to provide you with suggestions about the quality of probiotics that they carry.

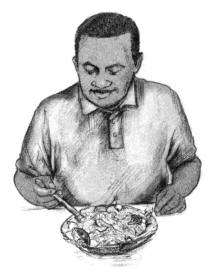

Fermented foods are the best to add natural probiotics and many other benefits, such as vitamins and minerals. Health food stores now carry a variety of fermented foods to choose from. Fermenting foods on your own is not only easy, but it is also very cost effective. And a big bonus is that it doesn't have to take up much space. It is very doable in the truck. You can ferment cabbage, any vegetable, fruit, or meat that you choose, in a quart jar. In some cases it is done in just a few days. The important thing to remember is that it needs to be raw and unpasteurized to have the live probiotics and enzymes that it needs to make it so beneficial. If it is heated, it will kill off all the necessary microorganisms needed to replenish the gut. If you haven't tried fermented foods, I challenge you to do so. You just might be pleasantly surprised. A friend of mine fermented some cucumbers in quart jars and they were the best dill pickles that I have ever eaten in my life. By adding fermented foods and probiotics to your routine, you will jump start your journey to good gut health, which can lead to overall good health.

Another gut health booster is bone broth. If you haven't already heard of this, it is made by cooking bones and other animal parts slowly in water. The easiest way is in the crock pot. When I first learned of this I thought where in the world do I get bones? I was surprised to find that most places that cut meat will also carry bones, BUT be sure that they are organically raised. It is very simple to do by placing the bones and other parts into the pot and adding water. That's it! Cook for 24 to 48 hours, and it is done.

There are many tutorials on the internet that can give you visual detail on how to do it. The reason bone broth works is that it has many nutrients in-

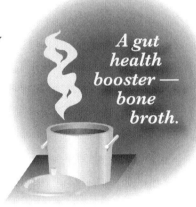

A gut health booster — bone broth.

cluding glucosamine and chondroitin. These substances help to heal the gut by sealing the enlarged holes that may be present due to bad eating habits, medications, stress, and so on. It works much like the product that you add to your tires that seals the holes in them. It also helps with joint pain and inflammation, while nourishing the bones, skin, hair, and nails; it may even fight infection. No wonder Grandma's homemade chicken soup made us feel so much better.

To add even more punch to the healing qualities add some herbs and vegetables to the pot. Each herb has different healing qualities. If this interests you, read up on the wonderful blessings that herbs have to offer our well being. Garlic and onion are great additions to healing too. You can find broths in the store, but making it homemade will cut down on the cost. Since it is easy to make in the crock pot if you have a way to keep it secure, you could make this in the truck too. If you are buying premade broth, be sure to watch for MSG and sugars. If at all possible, GO ORGANIC.

I hope that after reading this book you will know which kinds of foods lift us up and which bring us down. Which ones are beneficial to our gut, and which ones are not? Are you thinking, "What can I eat?" Don't worry. This book will open up a new world to the delicious, nutritious foods that are available. Healthy guts, healthy life, feeling great, here we come!

Endnotes

[1] Eveleth, Rose. (2013 October 24). "There are 37.2 Trillion Cells in Your Body." http://www/smithsonianmag.com/smart-news/there-are-372-trillion-cells-in-your-body-49 41473/?no-ist

[2] Greshko, Michael. (2016 January 13). "How Many Cells Are in the Human Body—And How Many Microbes?" http://news.nationalgeographic.com/2016/01/160111-microbiome-estimate-cout-ration-human-health-science/

[3] (2016 JApril 25) http://www.yeastconnection.com/pdf/DailySymptom-Chart.pdf

[4] Richards, Lisa. (2016 April 25) "Candida Symptoms" http://www.the candidadiet.com/candidasymptoms.htm

Thoughts to Ponder

1. What is the most interesting thing you have discovered about how your gut works?

2. What have you committed to do about improving your gut health?

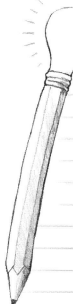

3. What is the first thing that you
   will change?

4. How does stress affect your life?

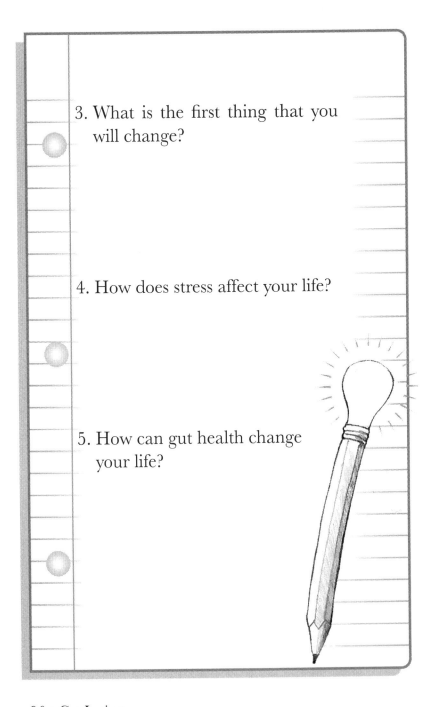

5. How can gut health change
   your life?

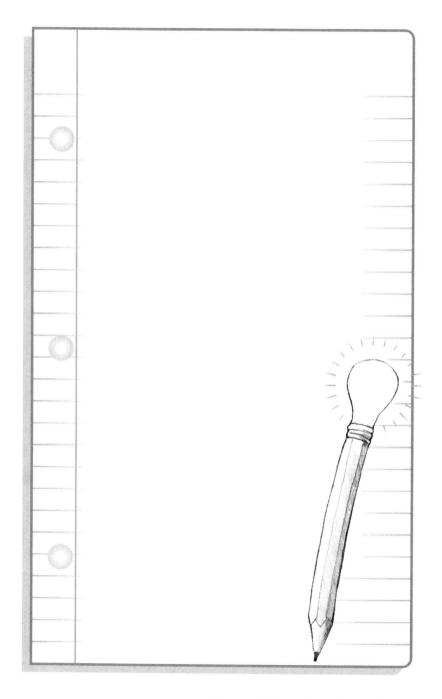

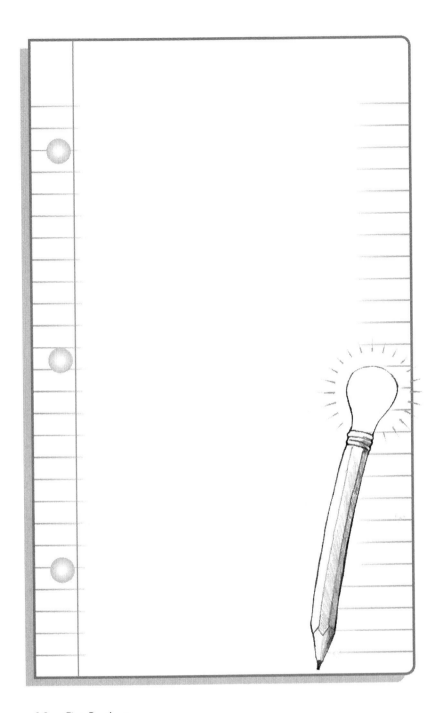

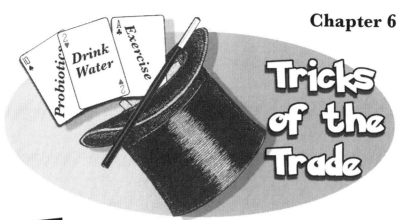

Chapter 6

Tricks of the Trade

Tricks of the trade: These have worked for me, and some of these I never want to be without.

Acid reflux –

probiotics, apple cider vinegar, or HCL capsules. This and eating right has stopped acid reflux in its tracks for me.

Upset stomach –

activated charcoal capsules, peppermint tea, probiotics, lemon, (*Important note:* When I took activated charcoal, my stool was black; this is ok. If stool is black and charcoal is not being taken, go to the doctor.)

Constipation –

WATER, eating right, probiotics, vitamin C flush, magnesium, fresh pears or green apples on an empty stomach, warm water and fresh squeezed lemon first thing in the morning at least thirty minutes before eating, exercise, prunes, prune juice, ground flax, a good quality olive oil with some fresh squeezed lemon on an empty stomach. If you're in the convenience of home, use an enema.

Diarrhea –

Drink WATER... One thing that I learned the hard way is that it is not always best to stop diarrhea. If there is diarrhea because it's getting rid of a virus or bacteria or some form of food poisoning or intruder, I will let it be. If I am over the issue, and it is just still there because it seems to have forgotten to go back to normal, here are my tricks: probiotics, bananas, rice, and tea made with fresh ginger seem to soothe it.

To cover it all, exercise.

Exercise gets things moving and steady. It seems like a simple suggestion, but it is essential. All the functions of our body are designed to work best with movement that has resistance. I know it is more difficult to find the time and means to get out there and move when you drive a truck for so many hours a day, but where there is a will there is a way, driver. Put exercise in your day as much as possible; your body will thank you with better health. You can do it!

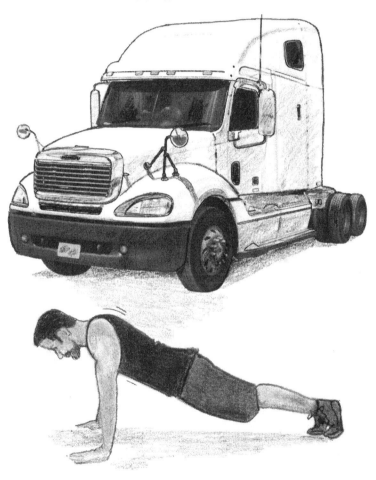

Thoughts to Ponder

1. What natural things do you already use to help with keeping healthy?

2. What natural health alternatives are interesting to you?

3. What things that are unnatural can you replace with natural?

4. What natural idea has helped you the most?

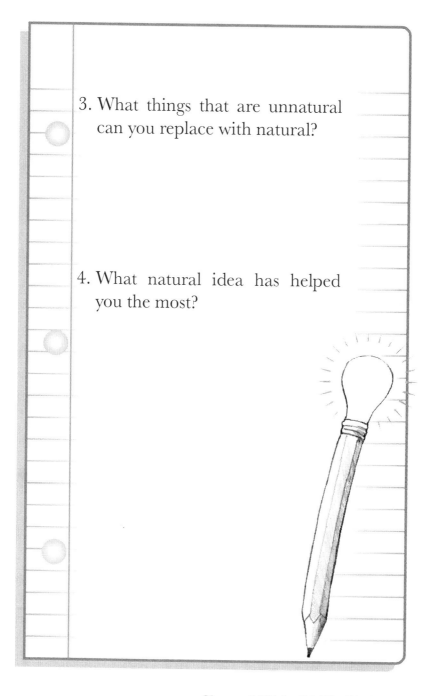

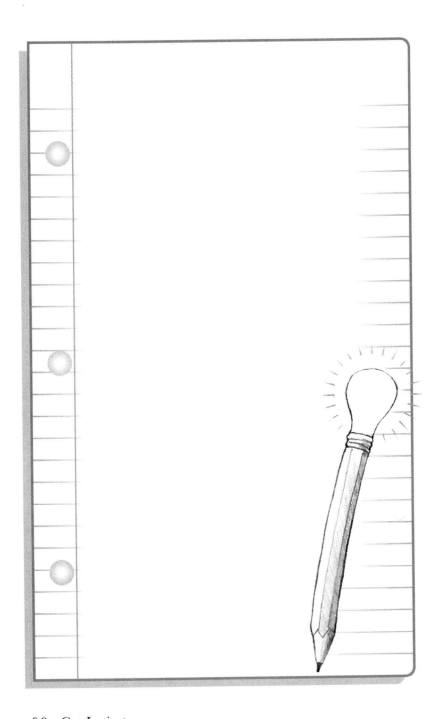

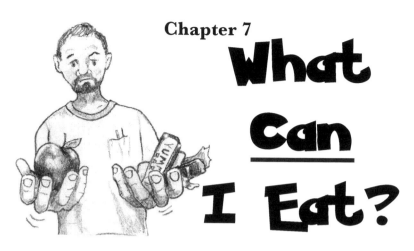

Chapter 7
What Can I Eat?

"One should eat to live, not live to eat."
—Benjamin Franklin

With this long list of foods, let's get your creativity going. Turn on the tube to a healthy channel for some ideas. Buy some recipe books. Look up recipes on the Internet that have the ingredients that you have on hand or that you are wanting to try out. With unlimited access to the Internet there is an endless supply of ideas for meals that are healthy and delicious. Get on social media and join a group that eats healthy on the road like Heart Smart Highway. Subscribe to sites that send free blog emails with healthy ideas, for example www.lifecoachservice.net.

YOU CAN DO THIS!!!!
I KNOW YOU CAN!!!!

Look for teas that have only the herb/herbs as the ingredient with no additives. Not only are these teas nourishing, many of them have healing qualities. I have never experienced a negative reaction with these teas, but if you have a medical situation or are on medication, I would do some research first to be sure.

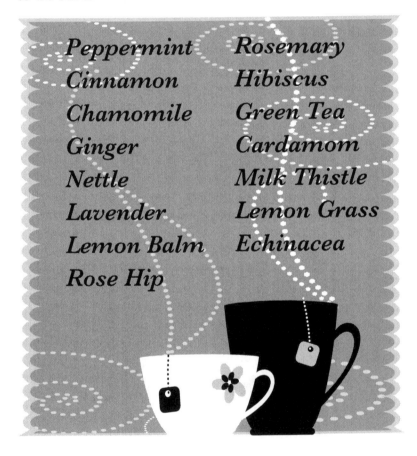

Peppermint   *Rosemary*
Cinnamon   *Hibiscus*
Chamomile   *Green Tea*
Ginger   *Cardamom*
Nettle   *Milk Thistle*
Lavender   *Lemon Grass*
Lemon Balm   *Echinacea*
Rose Hip

~ Vegetables ~

I personally have never met a vegetable that I didn't like, but many people don't have this outlook on vegetables. This list will give you a few ideas to start out with. Don't limit yourself. There are many more vegetables available to use and to try. All raw vegetables or vegetables cooked without harmful additives are a green light. Try to get organic as much as possible.

Underline your favorites!
Put a check by the ones you want to try out.

☐ Artichoke   ☐ Arugula

☐ Asparagus   ☐ Avocado

☐ Bamboo Shoots   ☐ Bean Sprouts

☐ Beans   ☐ Beets

☐ Bell Pepper   ☐ Bok Choy

☐ Broccoli   ☐ Garlic

☐ Ginger   ☐ Grape Leaves

☐ Wax Beans   ☐ Greens (Beet Greens)

☐ Collard Greens   ☐ Dandelion Greens

- ☐ Kohlrabi Greens
- ☐ Spinach
- ☐ Turnip Greens
- ☐ Horseradish
- ☐ Kale
- ☐ Lemongrass
- ☐ Pumpkin
- ☐ Tomatillo
- ☐ Turnip
- ☐ Watercress
- ☐ Brussels Sprouts
- ☐ Carrot
- ☐ Celery
- ☐ Cucumbers
- ☐ Elephant Garlic
- ☐ Mushrooms

- ☐ Mustard Greens
- ☐ Swiss Chard
- ☐ Hearts Of Palm
- ☐ Jerusalem Artichoke
- ☐ Leeks
- ☐ Shallots
- ☐ Swiss Chard
- ☐ Tomato
- ☐ Water Chestnuts
- ☐ Zucchini
- ☐ Cabbage
- ☐ Cauliflower
- ☐ Chinese Broccoli
- ☐ Eggplant
- ☐ Fennel
- ☐ Okra

- [ ] Olives
- [ ] Radish
- [ ] Sea Vegetables
- [ ] Squash
- [ ] Parsley
- [ ] Green Peas
- [ ] Sugar Snap Peas
- [ ] Plantain
- [ ] Onions
- [ ] Rutabaga
- [ ] Spinach
- [ ] Sweet Potato
- [ ] Peas
- [ ] Snow Peas
- [ ] Peppers
- [ ] Potato
- [ ] Green Beans/String Beans/Snap Beans
- [ ] Green Onions/Scallions
- [ ] Lettuce (Iceberg, Green Leaf, Red Leaf, Romaine)

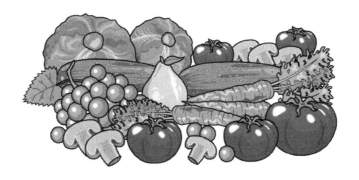

⎯ Fruits ⎯

The same rule goes for fruits. If they are in natural form, go for it!

☐ Apples

☐ Avocados

☐ Berries

☐ Coconuts

☐ Dates

☐ Melons

☐ Nonis

☐ Passion Fruits

☐ Pears

☐ Pineapples

☐ Grapes

☐ Guavas

☐ Kumquats

☐ Apricots

☐ Bananas

☐ Cherries

☐ Currants

☐ Figs

☐ Nectarines

☐ Papayas

☐ Peaches

☐ Persimmons

☐ Gingers

☐ Grapefruits

☐ Kiwis

☐ Lemons

☐ Limes   ☐ Mangos

☐ Mangosteens   ☐ Plantains

☐ Plums   ☐ Prunes

☐ Pomegranates   ☐ Prickly Pears

☐ Raisins   ☐ Rhubarbs

☐ Starfruits   ☐ Tangerines

☐ Tangelos   ☐ Tomatoes

☐ Oranges (Blood Oranges, Mandarins, Clementines, Satsumas, Navels, Sevilles, Valencias)

～ Grains ～

If you are serious about healing your gut and love the idea of losing weight, staying away from all grains will guide you to that destination. If you choose to stay on grains, here is a list of the ones that are best for optimal nutrition. Eating them when sprouted is a plus. Ezekiel is a brand that has sprouted grain bread and is available for purchase in many stores.

Organic brown rice   Organic non-GMO corn
Organic oats   Organic rye
Organic stone-ground wheat

Grain Alternatives

Almond flour –
> This makes the BEST muffins in addition to many other things.

Chick pea flour –
> What I have used this for mostly is in making Indian dishes, but there are many other uses. We love it.

Coconut flour –
> This flour makes good pancakes and desserts. I used it to batter some fish once and it was good.

Quinoa –
> You can use this just like you would use rice. My family prefers it over rice.

Sunflower seed flour –
> I have eaten bread made with this, and it is good.

Sugars

Remember, we don't need much sugar at all. On those rare occasions that we want to give ourselves a treat, use these options.

This is a list of sugars that are minimally processed and have nutritional value.

•Coconut sugar •Date sugar
•Honey •Maple syrup

When wanting to sweeten something up, consider using fruit. I enjoy adding a banana to a smoothie, and it is plenty sweet.

—∿— Meats —∿—

Keep in mind how these meats are processed. Sometimes it is difficult to find quality meats. I have found that most people eat much more meat than what is necessary for good health. If you choose to eat meat, be sure to be very picky. Here is a checklist of things to look for when buying quality meat:

• Was it raised free range?

• Was it raised organically?

• Was it fed anything that this animal was not designed to eat, such as vegetarian-fed chicken? Chickens are not vegetarians.

• Was it fed GMOs?

These are common meats that can be healthy if they meet the above specifications.

Beef	Deer	Pheasant
Buffalo	Chicken	Quail
Lamb	Duck	Turkey
Moose	Goose	Eggs

Albacore tuna from the U.S. or British Columbia

Dungeness crab, wild caught

Mussels farmed in the U.S.

Salmon - wild caught Alaska

Oysters farmed

Rainbow trout farmed in the U.S.

Sardines wild caught pacific

—Spices—

Spices are not only yummy to the tummy, but they are also nutritional and healing. Again, always look for organic if possible. Beware of spices from other countries, some may be fine and some not. Do the research. Here is a good start for you.

Allspice, ground and whole

Arrowroot starch

Basil

Bay leaves

Chili powder

Cinnamon, ground and sticks

Cloves, ground and whole

Coriander, ground

Cumin, ground

Curry powder

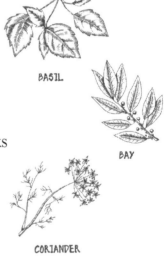

BASIL

BAY

CORIANDER

Dill weed
Fennel seeds
Five-spice powder
Garlic powder
Ginger, ground
Marjoram, dried
Mint, dried
Mustard, dried ground
Nutmeg
Onion powder
Oregano, dried
Paprika, Hungarian sweet
Pepper, cayenne, dried red flakes
Peppermint
Peppercorns, dried black
Poppy seeds
Rosemary, dried
Sage, dried and rubbed
Salt, table and Kosher
Sesame seeds
Tarragon, dried
Thyme, ground and dried
Turmeric
Vanilla extract

FENNEL

GINGER

MINT

MUSTARD

NUTMEG

OREGANO

ROSEMARY

THYME

SAGE

Thoughts to Ponder

1. Which statement describes your habits: eat to live or live to eat?

2. What are your favorite vegetables?

3. Which ones that you have just discovered will you try first?

4. How much driving force are you willing to provide for making healthy decisions?

5. What new choices do you feel you have now?

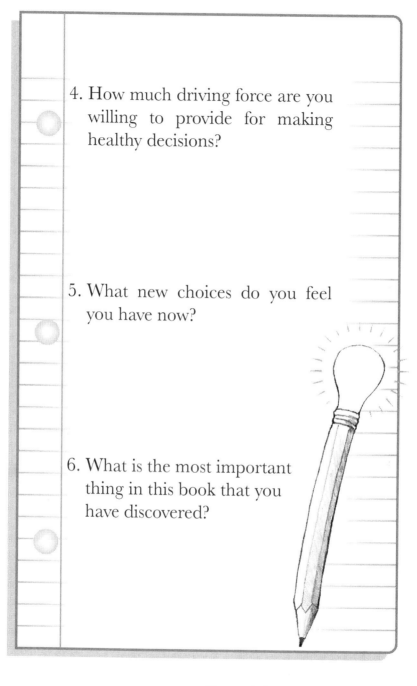

6. What is the most important thing in this book that you have discovered?

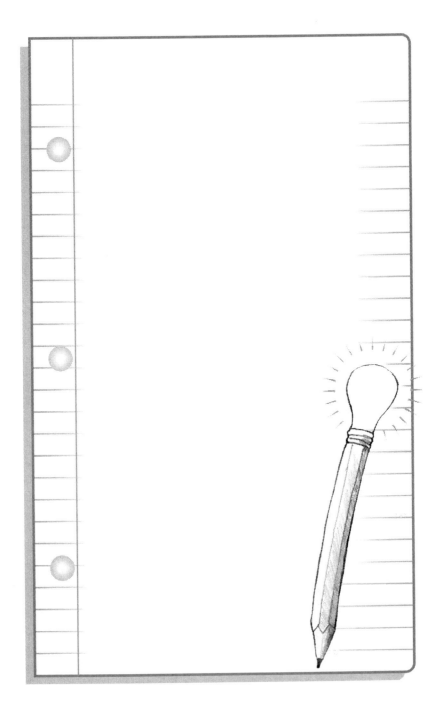

Chapter 8

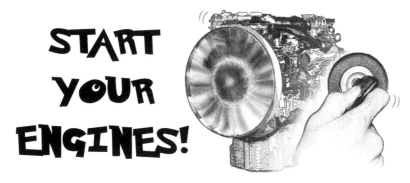

START YOUR ENGINES!

T he biggest part of success is to MAKE A PLAN!!!!

If you don't make a plan, it will be hard for you to have success. It also saves lots of time and money.

You now have enough information to set yourself in the right direction. At first some of these ideas and products may be very new to you, but this will change. As you begin your journey into health you will discover a new world of foods and solutions that have always been there but you were not aware of. Just as it gets easier and more familiar the more times you go down the same road, you will find the road

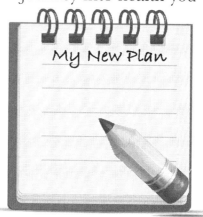

to better health gets easier with practice. This life change will get easier and more comfortable as you learn and explore this new journey to health. Adjust this newfound information in a way that will work the best for you.

Some will take this information, run with it and never look back. Others will take it and form it to suit their way of changing things in their lives by taking baby steps. Either way, don't let bumps in

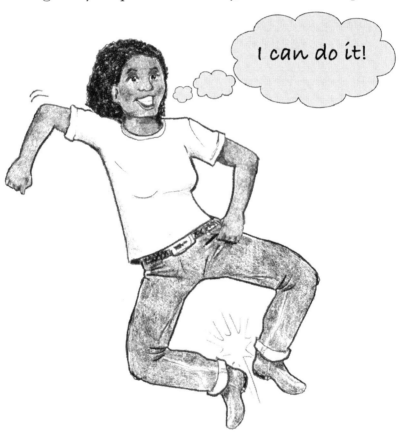

the road veer you off track. Look ahead, keep your eye on the goal, and press on, driver.

I want these recipes to serve as the beginning of your creativity and excitement of food - good, healthy food. I have also selected these recipes not only to be healthy but to be very easy. When you step over into the threshold of health, you will look at the old way of eating in a completely different way. The feelings of being deprived of the old foods will lessen. These past substances appear to be food, but in reality they are a mixture of things that have no nutritional value and shouldn't even be considered food at all. Your body will feel so marvelous and vibrant that eating the old way will not be worth the tradeoff of this great and healthful feeling. Keep in mind, though, that it takes a month or so for your stomach to get out of the habit of feeling the need for so much food. When the toxins have stopped going into your body, they will not be reminding you to want more. It is a change of habit that will be faster for some and slower for others. Either way, the courage and persistence is very worth it.

Some of these foods might be unfamiliar to you. Not too many years ago, it might have been hard to find them, but now you should be able to find them at your local grocery store. Don't let the fact that they are unfamiliar keep you from trying them. Be adventurous! I have also added some ideas to try when you are home to take back out on the road.

Just because some of these foods are traditionally eaten at certain times of the day doesn't mean you can't eat them at other times. Don't limit yourself. You can have a smoothie for supper and leftovers for breakfast. Lots of times drivers work, eat, and sleep at different times of the day than most people, anyway. Get creative with the food choices that you put together.

I have put these recipes in a format that will enable you to go to one section and pick from something there and go to another section to add to it to make a meal. This will open up the possibilities to much more variety on the plate. For example, go to the meal starter section and pick something from there. It may need a couple of vegetables to go with it. Then go to the veggie section to pick from there.

For meat eaters, as I mentioned already, be very picky about the meat that you buy. Be sure that it is grass-fed organic or free-range organic. If you are having a hard time finding it, it's ok to skip the meat altogether until you can find a good source. Keep looking, it is there.

Cooking oil – Are you already choosing the right cooking oil? Cooking oils are not all created equal. Many of them are very processed and a GMO (genetically modified organism). Cooking this wonderfully nutritious food in an oil that can be detrimental to your health will defeat the purpose of eating healthy. Be very picky when choosing cooking oil. Look for organic and not processed.

Coconut oil is the most versatile and healthy choice. Choose organic extra virgin cold pressed. This can be used as a cooking oil, a spread, skin moisturizer, medicine for cuts and scrapes, and it is wonderful for dental hygiene.

Olive oil is also good as long as it is not cooked at high temperatures and is of a good quality. Extra virgin olive oil has more health benefits than regular olive oil. This can also be used as a skin moisturizer and on cuts and scrapes.

Sunflower oil and *avocado oil* are not as widely known, but they are also a healthy choice. Vegetable oils and canola oils are most likely GMO and do not promote health. Anything hydrogenated (made into a solid) will also have negative health effects.

You will notice that I mention the crock pot quite often. This is because I have more experience with it than the others. It does not mean that you have to have and use a crock pot or that it is the only way to cook in the truck. Don't limit yourself. There are many choices. Of course you have to have something to cook in, but as you will read in a moment, there are so many options to choose from.

Many of these small appliances have recipes that come with them.

Mentioned below are some small appliances that will make healthy eating very doable in the truck.

—ᴡᴡ— Appliances —ᴡᴡ—

Inverter

Refrigerator or some kind of cooler
to keep foods cold

Freezer

Crock pot/slow cooker

Personal size blender

Toaster oven

Rice cooker

Single or double eye cooktop

Wok

Gas grill

Lunch box

Nuwave grill

Toaster

Aroma cooker

Hot plate

George Foreman grill

Aroma electric skillet

Ninja 3 in one cooker

Induction burner

Convection oven

Percolator

Pizza oven

Griddle

Hot air popper

Mini food chopper

Hand mixer

Sandwich maker

Blender

Mandolin slicer

Egg cooker

Rocket grill

Little smoky joe BBQ grill

Single burner butane stove

Keurig mini

French press

Indoor grill

12 volt oven

Rice cooker

I looked up twelve volt appliances on the internet. There are many choices available. If you have some tricks of the trade that make food preparation in the truck more convenient that you may already use, send me an email. I'd like to know! Give me your feedback at info@lifecoachservice.net.

Easy And Healthy Foods Always To Have On Hand

A wonderful thing about raw whole foods is that many of them need no refrigeration, like fruits and root vegetables. This can give you an abundance of choices and more room in the fridge for other things.

Some of you can buy most of your produce when you are home and wash them all before you leave. Then they are ready to eat when the time comes.

You can make your greens last longer for smoothies, and save money, by freezing them and just take out how much you need each time.

Some of the foods that are high in nutrients yet unfamiliar might be as follows:

*Challenge

Look up the nutrition values of these foods. You will want to put them in every-thing!.

Chia seed - this is a highly nutritious seed that helps with weight loss and keeps you full longer. It also has omega 3. Not only is this really good in smoothies, it is good sprinkled on salads and other foods. Be sure to have liquids with this, as chia seeds absorb a huge amount.

> ***Chia and hemp and flax can be added to any smoothie or sprinkled on any meal for added benefit.***

Hemp seed – (Be sure it says hemp seed and not hemp powder.) This seed is high in protein and has many other nutritional values. For a mid-day pick me up, find a way to add this to what you are eating. You can put this in any smoothie, sprinkle it on a salad or on the food that you are eating.

Flax seed – always make sure that flax seed is going to be ground up when you are eating it. The outer part of the seed will not digest and will be of no benefit. It also has omega 3 and is a very good fiber. It can also be added to any smoothie and sprinkled on foods. It is very good when added to muffins.

Coconut sugar – The name says it all. Sweet brown granules from the coconut. It reminds me of brown sugar.

Date Sugar – this is ground up dates. It has a very nice flavor.

Think of a recipe as a compass not a map!

Happy eating!

Thoughts to Ponder

1. What eating plan are you currently using?

2. What are you going to change about your plan?

3. How does it make you feel when you create?

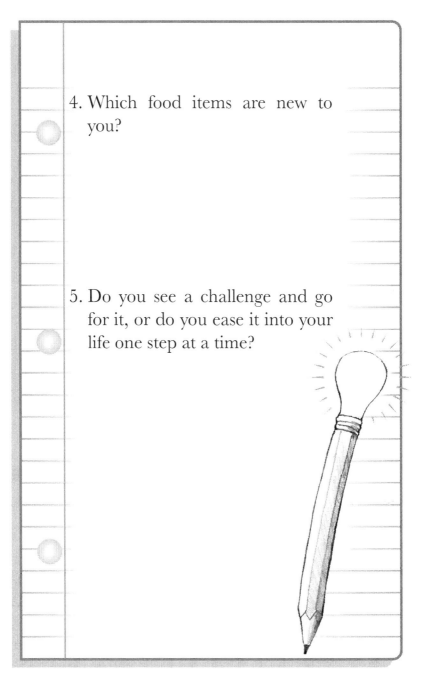

4. Which food items are new to you?

5. Do you see a challenge and go for it, or do you ease it into your life one step at a time?

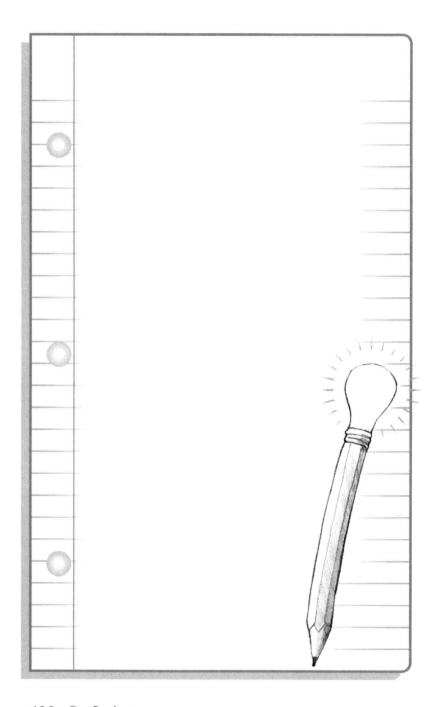

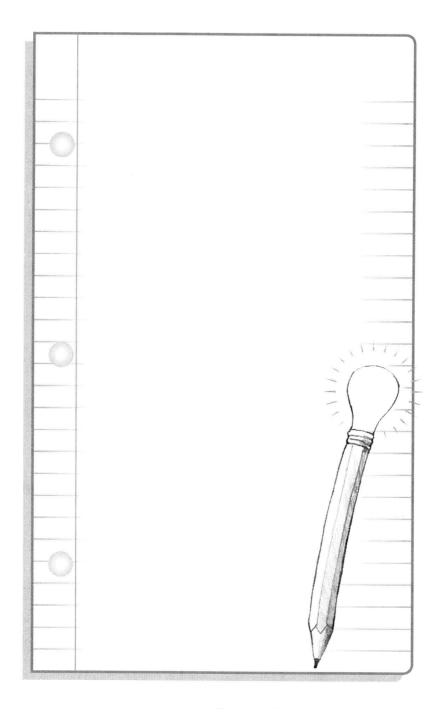

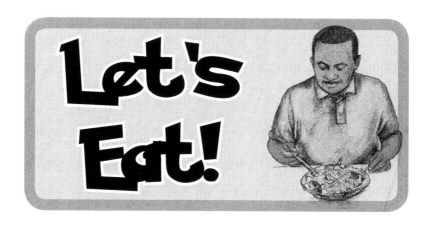

5 Day Sample Menu Plan

This example is just to show you some ideas on how a healthy meal plan looks. Use this plan as a starter to get creative ideas flowing in your mind. Try new things. Use the healthy foods that you like. As you come up with your own ideas, write them down in the spaces provided. It's your choice. Will you choose healthy? It's your plan that determines the road to health and wellness.

Remember, as your meal schedule changes from day to day, these eating arrangements can interchange at different times of the day. If possible, try to eat less at night.

Day One

Breakfast
Strawberry banana smoothie

Snack
Carrot sticks dipped in guacamole

Lunch
Garden salad with a boiled egg

Supper
Plan ahead if you have only one source of cooking.
Meat loaf   Sweet potatoes
Green beans

Day Two

Breakfast
Sliced apple and almond butter or sun butter

Snack
Granola

Lunch
Salmon salad

Supper
Lentil soup

Day 3
Breakfast
Blueberry peach smoothie
Snack
*(A healthy dessert that is so good for you,
it can be a snack or a meal)*
Chocolate pudding
Lunch
Broccoli salad
Supper
Roast with carrots, and onions
Butter beans
Greens

Day 4
Breakfast
Banana and almond butter or sun butter
Snack
Buffalo cauliflower
Lunch
Baby carrots, celery and/or cucumber slices
dipped in hummus
Supper
Use the leftover roast from the day before,
add BBQ sauce, with roasted vegetables on
the side.

Day 5
Breakfast
Granola
Snack
Strawberries
Lunch
Avocado tuna salad
Supper
Chili

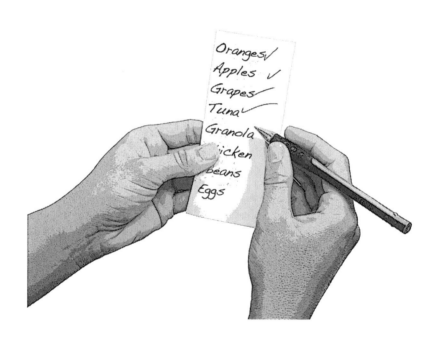

⎯ᴡ⎯Smoothies⎯ᴡ⎯

All of these smoothies can be altered to your taste. Add a little of this and take a little of that. Some blenders require more water to make them blend; if that's the case, they will not be as thick but that's ok. If you like smoothies colder, add ice.

With smoothies the sky's the limit.

Here are some to base your creativity on and learn which flavors suit you best. From there just dump some goodies in and blend. You're the chef! For the most part, smoothies consist of a **liquid** such as water or a nut or seed milk like coconut milk, almond milk or hemp milk. **Fruit** such as berries, melons and bananas. **Some extra nutrition** such as hemp seed, chia, nuts, avocado, and greens (spinach and kale).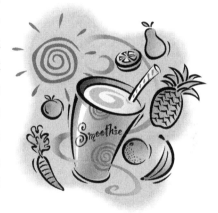

For those of you who don't like avocado, put an avocado in your smoothie, you'll never know it's there. Same goes for greens; start with spinach. It takes quite a bit of spinach to even know that there is a green in there. Just don't be intimidated by the color. It is the taste and nutrition that we are going for. If you put strawberries and greens together such as spinach, the color will not be pretty and pink. That is ok! This is an awesome way to get the nutrients into your body that it truly needs.

Spinach Mango

1 mango	Some spinach (a handful)
1 orange	About ¾ cup of water
1 banana	

Peel fruit, cut into pieces that fit into your blender and blend.

Apple Strawberry

1 cup fresh or frozen strawberries

1 apple

1-2 cups of greens

Give or take a cup of water

Take green tops off strawberries, slice and core the apple, throw in the greens and water and blend.

Avocado Chocolate Almond Butter

½ ripe avocado

1 frozen banana

2 T cocoa powder

3 T almond butter

1½ cups almond milk

A natural sweetener to taste

Blend

Mandarin Orange

(Do you remember pushups popsicles?)

½ banana

2 mandarin oranges

4 or more ice cubes

1 cup almond milk unsweetened

1 t pure vanilla extract

Peel all fruit, dump it all in and blend

Strawberry Banana

2 cups of frozen strawberries

1 banana

1 cup or so of water or almond milk

Peel, add, and blend

Orange Mango

1 orange

1 mango

1 cup of frozen strawberries

1 cup or so of water or almond milk

Peel, add, and blend

Apple Kale Avocado

1 avocado

1 green apple cored and diced

1 cup kale

1 banana

1 cup of water or almond milk

Peel fruit; add and blend

Grapefruit Kale

1 cup ice   1 grapefruit

1 banana   3 cups kale

½ cup pineapple

Peel fruits. Add everything but the ice. Blend really well. Add ice, and blend again.

Purple

1 banana

½ cup of frozen mixed berries or blueberries

2 cups of kale

1 cup or so of water

Add and blend.

Supper Food

2 cups cold water	½ cored chopped apple
1 cup spinach	Juice of ½ lemon
1 leaf kale	1 cucumber

Add and blend

Green Lemonade

1 pear cored and sliced

1 cucumber cut into pieces

Juice of ½ lemon

2 cups kale

¾ cup or so of water

¼ cup ice

Add and blend

Blueberry Peach

2 cups frozen blueberries

1 cup frozen or fresh peach

1 banana

1 T chia

1 cup kale

1 to 2 cups of water

Add and blend.

Green Pear

3 ripe pears cored and sliced

½ cup pineapple

1 cup kale

1 cup or so of water

Add a banana or not

Add and blend

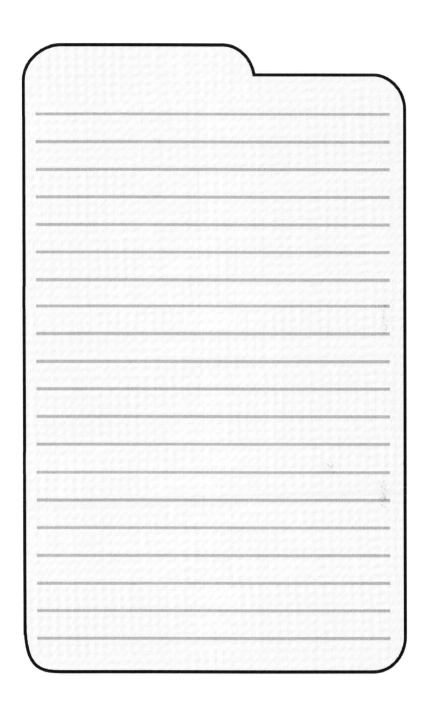

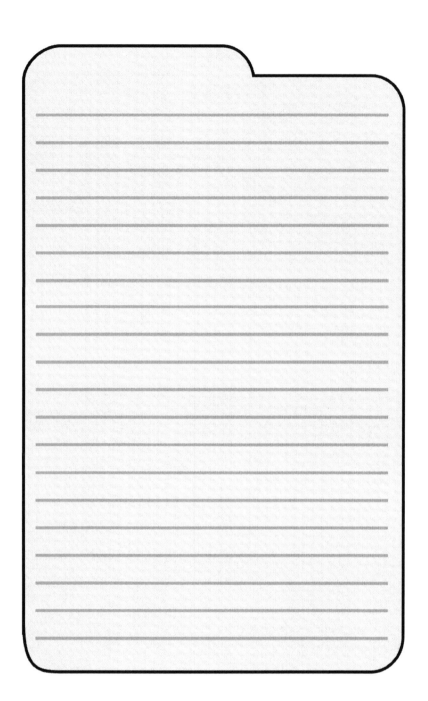

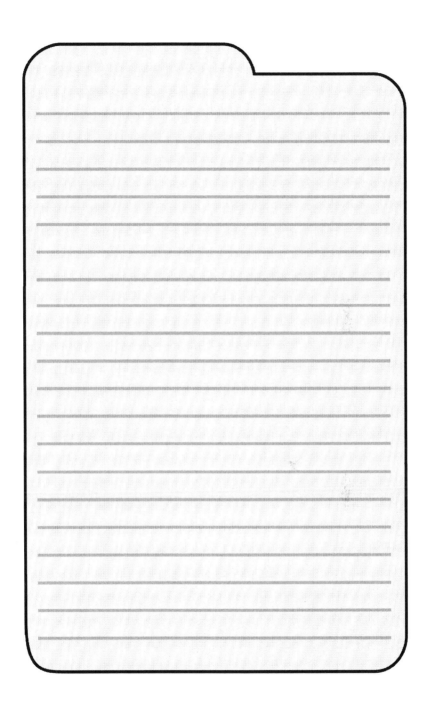

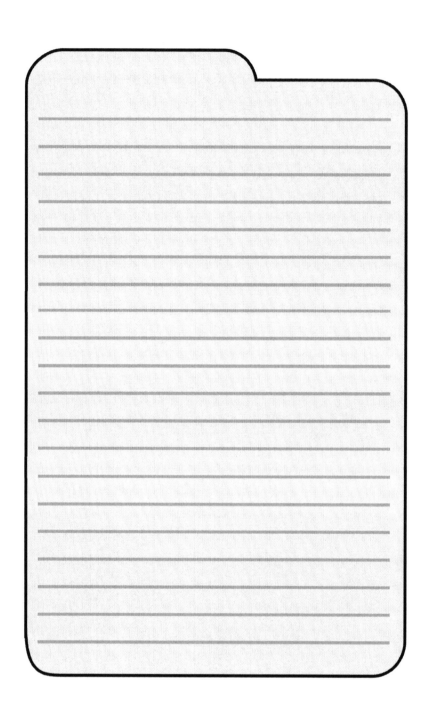

⋙—Snacks—⋘

First go back to the page with the list of "what I can eat" foods. There's a long list of fruits and vegetables that will be perfect for snacks. As with all other recipes, make a plan. Make a meal chart, see what items that you need for it, and buy them at the grocery store. Then make time for some prep work so that when it is time to eat throughout the week, there it is all ready to eat. Put snacks in individual containers or baggies, so that you can portion control. Simple is good.

Carrot sticks

Celery and almond butter/sun butter

Apples and almond butter/sun butter

Chopped melon in a cup

Any kind of chopped fruit covered in nuts such as walnuts, pecans, or almonds

Frozen blueberries

Banana almond butter/sun butter

Avocado with salt on it

Raisins/currants

Fresh strawberries and bananas

Pumpkin seeds

Oranges

Bananas

Grapefruits

Grapes

Strawberries

Blueberries

Blackberries

Raspberries

Cherries

Papaya

All melons

Pineapples

Mangos

Sunflower seeds

All fresh fruit

Apples

Pears

Plums

Grapes

Unsweetened large flaked coconut

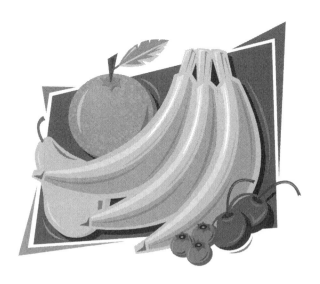

Boiled Egg

In rice cooker - Add the water to the inner pot of your rice cooker. Place eggs in the steam tray and set to steam for 10-15 minutes, depending how you like your eggs.

In crock pot – Place eggs in crock pot, with enough water to cover them. Put the lid on and set on high 2 ½ hours.

You can eat them just plain, make deviled eggs, add them to salad, or make egg salad.

Homemade Granola

1 cup raw pumpkin seeds

1 cup raw sunflower seeds

1 cup unsweetened coconut flakes

1 cup raw sliced almonds

2 cups pecans

20 dates chopped finely

1/3 cup coconut oil

2 t cinnamon

3 t vanilla

A dash of salt

If you leave out the coconut oil, cinnamon, salt, and vanilla, you won't have to cook it and, it is done. If you want it roasted with some flavor, mix all the ingredients together well. In any cooker that will hold it, cook until done. Cook it in an oven at 325 degrees for 20 minutes. If you're using a crock pot, cook it on low for 2 to 3 hours. Warning, the smell is going to torture you.

Herbed Almonds

2 cups of raw almonds

½ t black pepper

½ t salt

1 T dried thyme

1 T rosemary

1 T olive oil

Combine and cook on high, in a crock pot, for 1 ½ hours stirring every 30 minutes. Serve warm or cold. (Try some garlic with this too.)

Guacamole

Start with one ripe avocado and add any of the following:

Chopped onions

Chopped tomatoes

Lemon juice

Salt

Jalapeños

Salsa

Mash avocado, add ingredients, and mix well. Get creative!

You could use carrots or celery, sliced bell peppers, broccoli, cauliflower, or spread it on romaine lettuce leaves and roll up for a yummy roll up.

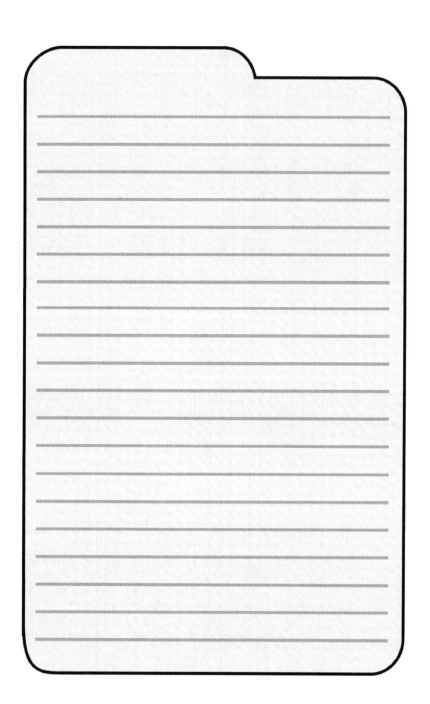

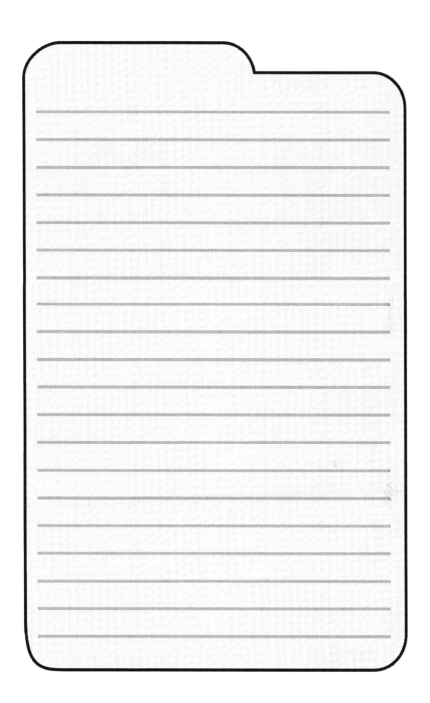

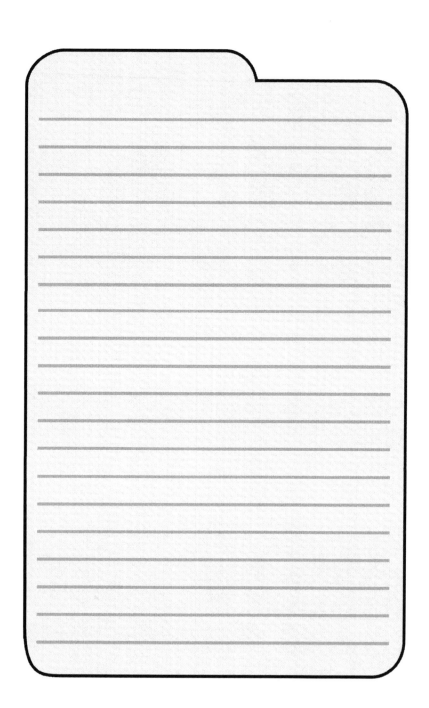

⚬⚬⚬ Dressings ⚬⚬⚬

Please take a very important note here. Store-bought dressings are NOT healthy. Homemade is so simple and fast.

French Dressing

1 squirt of mustard

1 Tablespoon tomato paste (organic)

1/3 cup olive oil

1/4 cup white wine vinegar

1 Tablespoon of honey (optional)

1/2 t onion powder or small chunk of fresh onion

Blend or whisk together.

Cilantro Dressing

1 cup chopped cilantro, stems removed

½ avocado

2 T fresh lime or lemon juice

1-2 cloves of garlic

¼ cup olive oil

2 t apple cider vinegar

1/8 t salt

½ t ground turmeric

Optional 1 t honey

Blend until smooth.

Ranch Dressing

½ cup sunflower seeds

1 cup coconut milk (canned, not the lite version, save any left over to put in a smoothie)

½ T onion powder

½ T garlic powder

½ t dill

1 t or less salt

A dash of pepper

Blend ingredients. This dressing is good instantly, but it will thicken and blend flavors if refrigerated overnight. I could add this to anything!!!

To make **chipotle dressing**, just add some hot sauce to this recipe and it is a magical transformation.

Avocado Ranch

1 avocado

1 cup almond, coconut, hemp, or cashew milk

3 T fresh lemon juice

1-2 cloves of garlic

½ t dill

½ t onion powder

Salt to taste

Dash of pepper

Blend

Greek Vinaigrette

¼ cup extra virgin olive oil

2 T red wine vinegar or apple cider vinegar

1 lemon juiced

2 cloves garlic minced

1 t oregano

Salt and pepper to taste

Add to jar and shake or whisk in bowl. The longer it sits the stronger the flavor. So if you like it mild, eat it soon. If you like it strong, like me, let it sit.

Orange Basil Vinaigrette

½ cup sunflower seeds

1 T mustard

2 T avocado oil

4 T orange juice or the juice of a orange

1 T apple cider vinegar

1 T honey

1 cup basil leaves

Blend

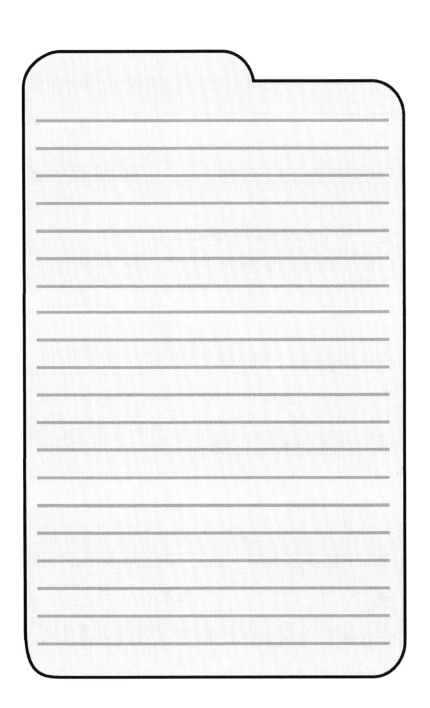

Get creative. Substitute one thing for another, or use what you have. Just think, you will have created a new favorite. And even better, most of the time, salad means NO COOKING!!!

Garden Salad

Yet another way to create. Take your choice of greens chopped or not, add bite size fresh vegetables, drizzle some healthy homemade dressing on it and voila! You are done!

Iceberg lettuce (a head of lettuce) has little nutritional value. Romaine lettuce is a good substitute. Also add kale, arugula, butterhead, chard, endive, escarole, leaf lettuce, radicchio, spinach, watercress, and even cabbage, as these have an abundance of nutrients. The more variety the more nutritional value.

Broccoli Salad

3 cups fresh broccoli chopped

½ cup of raisins, currants, or unsweetened dried cranberries, dried blueberries, or fresh pomegranate seeds

½ cup raw sunflower seeds

½ cup sliced almonds

½ onion diced small

1 T honey

2 T apple cider vinegar

1 T lemon juice

3 T olive oil

Salt and pepper to taste

Avocado Tuna Salad

1 avocado

1 lemon juiced

1 T chopped onion

1 can wild caught tuna

Salt and pepper to taste

Mix together tuna, lemon, onion, salt, pepper, stir well. Add diced avocado; mix well.

Just eat it like that with a spoon or place on a romaine lettuce leaf to make a roll up.

Southwest Salad
(one of my favorites!!!)

1 can black beans drained

1 bell pepper chopped, any color

½ cup chopped tomatoes

5 green onions chopped

1 chopped avocado

1 head of romaine lettuce chopped

This makes a lot of salad. Either reduce amounts for one person or keep ingredients separate and add them all to your bowl. Pop them back in the refrigerator and eat tomorrow. The best way to top this salad off is the cilantro or southwest dressing. YUM!

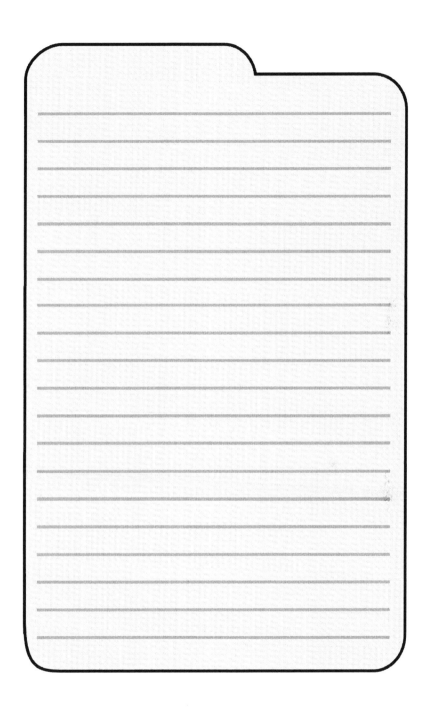

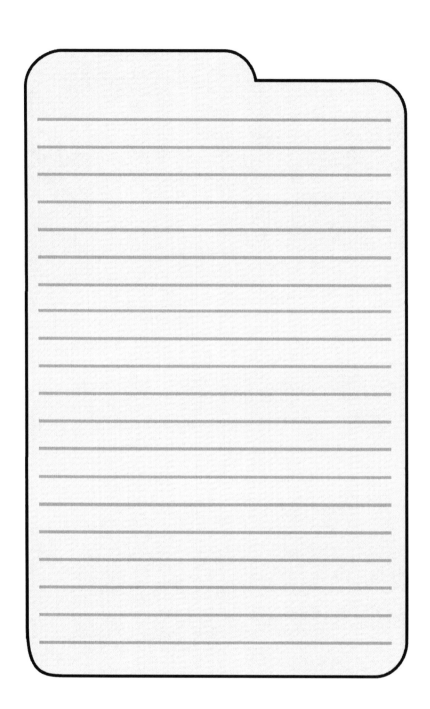

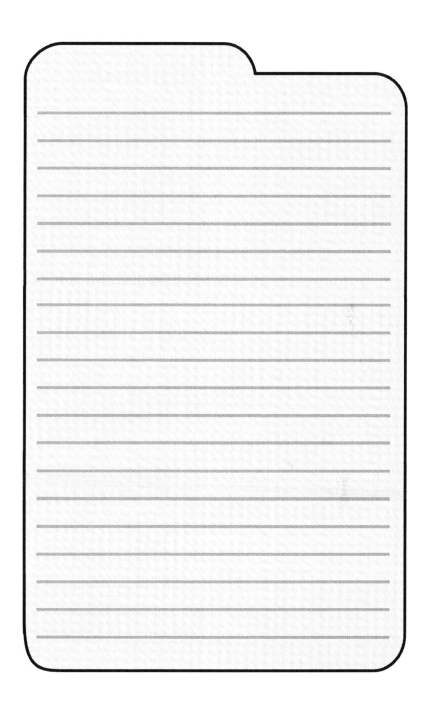

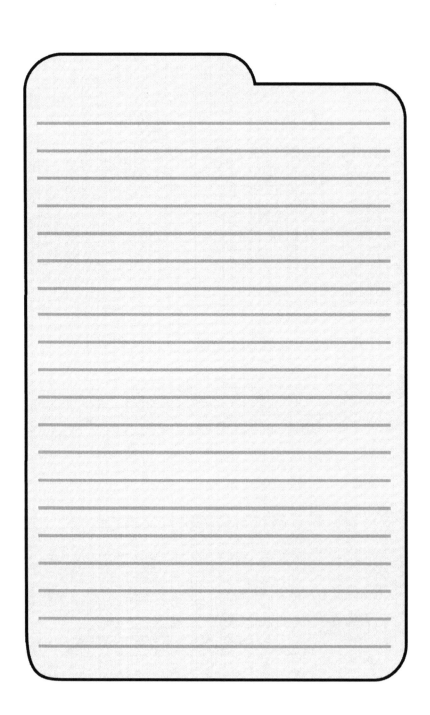

～— Vegetables —～

Vegetables can be as simple as one ingredient and a little salt or, they can get very elaborate. Either way, they are good. Just keep in mind to use fresh, all-natural ingredients, and you will be eating healthy and tantalizing your taste buds all at the same time.

Fresh is best, but frozen vegetables are a good way to add variety to any meal. You should be able to find these frozen vegetables at your local store. Just cook them up plain or spruce them up.

Lima beans

Butter beans

Carrots

Broccoli

Cauliflower

Green beans

Green peas

Snap peas

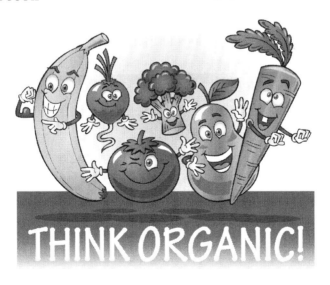

THINK ORGANIC!

Sweet Potato

The easiest and my favorite! Cook it peeling-on in the crock pot or any kind of heated appliance that will hold it and be covered. This usually takes a few hours. I like it when it cooks a little too long and sits a while. It makes it sweeter. This way, you don't need to add anything. It is good just the way it is. Of course adding some cinnamon really zings it up.

(You can do butternut squash this way too. When it is done just scrape out the seeds.)

Roasting Vegetables

This is the easiest way to get a variety of fresh vegetables that are oh-so-good. They all can be cooked at the same time and are good as leftovers.

Just spread them out on a sheet or put in your appliance of choice (This works in the crock pot.) add a healthy oil and seasonings and cook.

Some of my favorites to roast are, Brussels sprouts, green beans, carrots, onions, garlic, broccoli, cauliflower, snap peas and asparagus.

Roasted Green Beans

A bag of frozen whole green beans

Spread them out on a cookie sheet or in a pan that can bake

Drizzle coconut oil or olive oil over them

Sprinkle with your favorite herbs

Here are some herb ideas, Mrs. Dash, rosemary, cayenne, Italian seasoning, thyme, creole seasoning (Check for MSG), get creative.

Add salt and pepper

Bake at 350 degrees for 20-30 minutes. They will be done when they are soft and a little brown. One trick that I have found, if they are done, turn it off and just leave it for a while. It makes them even better. They are GREAT left over.

Carrots

Carrots can be used so many ways, including roasting or adding to soups. One way that my family enjoys carrots that I just made up one day, is to slice them to look like pennies, sauté them in coconut oil, when they are close to done, add salt and cayenne pepper.

Greens

Turnip, kale, spinach, mustard, collard

Add any greens to the crock pot. Add salt and cook. You can add seasoning, but they are good just as they are. Greens should be a part of every day for good health.

Buffalo Cauliflower

1 head of cauliflower chopped into bite-sized pieces

2 t organic garlic powder

Salt and pepper

1 T coconut oil

¾ cup of hot sauce

This can be a side dish or a good snack. Mix it all together, fully coating cauliflower. Oil pan with coconut oil. Cook at 450 degrees 20 minutes or until tender or in crock pot until tender.

Hummus
(OH, how I love hummus.)

You can make hummus out of any bean. I have also seen recipes using peas and cauliflower. It stores well and is typically very inexpensive to make.

The basic ingredients:

Chickpeas (Garbanzo beans are the same thing.)

Garlic

Lemon

Tahini

Olive oil

Although tahini really makes it have a great flavor, we have made it without when it wasn't available, and it was still good.

You can make it from canned beans, but what I have found is making it from dried beans and mixing it up while hot is the best way to make it really creamy. Either way will work just fine.

Different beans that you can use

Black	Pinto
Northern	Kidney

Some flavors to add to hummus:

Avocado	Rosemary
Roasted bell pepper	Sweet potato
Sundried tomato basil	Olive
Roasted garlic	Hot sauce
Sautéed onion	Jalapeno
Lemon	Lime cilantro
Kale	Spinach

Here's what to do

1 can of chickpeas

(or 1 ½ cup of dried chick peas cooked.)

1 clove of garlic

1 T organic extra virgin olive oil

½ cup of water or the liquid from the beans

Add it all to the blender, food processor, or personal blender and blend until very smooth. That's it!

Now what to dip it with? Baby carrots, cucumber slices, squash slices, celery, sliced bell peppers, broccoli, cauliflower, finger (LOL).

Sautéed Vegetables

You can sauté just about any vegetable that you wish. Just pick a healthy oil, gather some yummy herbs, and throw in some chopped vegetables at a medium heat and stir until they are as crunchy as you like. Salt and pepper and you are ready to eat.

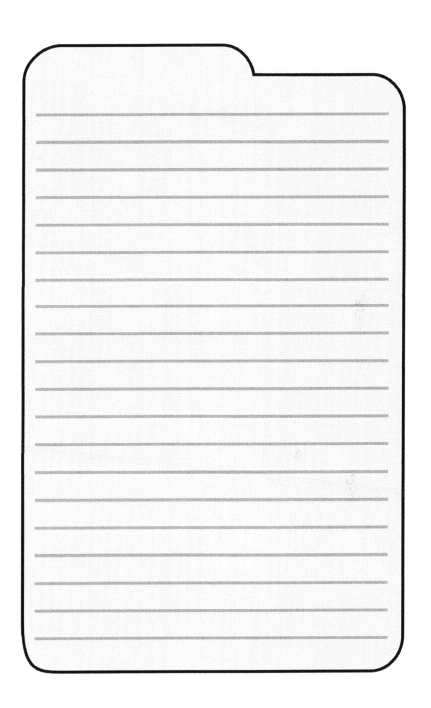

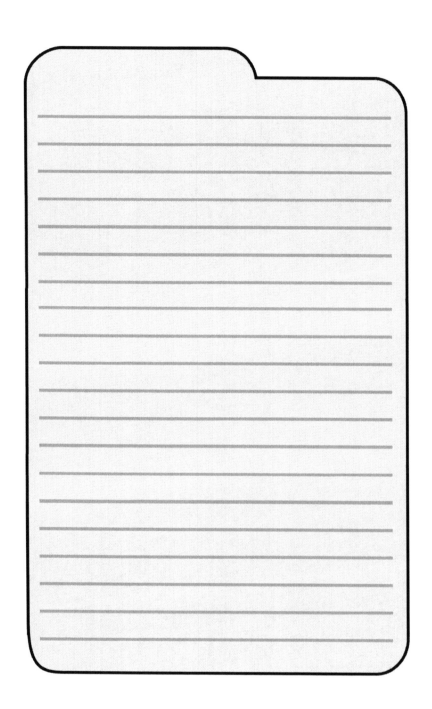

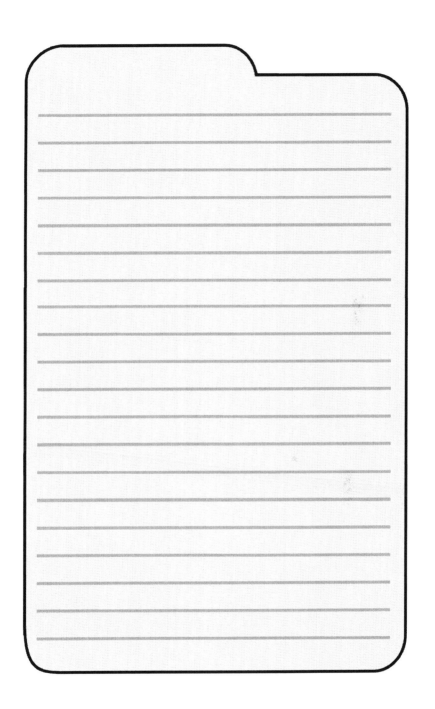

Meal Starters

Make two to three times as much meat for one meal; when it is done portion it out into three parts and then you can have easy meals for the next couple days. For instance if you make crock pot chicken and vegetables in the crock pot and eat one portion of the chicken and all the veggies, the next day you could dice the leftover chicken to make chicken salad or shred it up for BBQ chicken. Make freezer meals. Add the ingredients that you will need into a gallon size Ziplock bag and freeze. When you are ready to cook, have it partially thawed, and dump it all in. Voila! So easy.

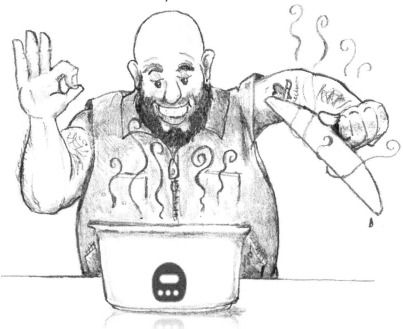

Lime Cilantro Chicken

3 chicken breasts

The juice from 2 limes

1 bunch of chopped cilantro

2 cloves of garlic

1 onion

1 can of beans of choice, drained

1 t cumin

1 t rosemary

Salt pepper

Add all ingredients and cook on low for 8 hours in the crock pot

Meatloaf
(in the crock pot)

1 pound of ground meat

1 chopped bell pepper

1 chopped onion

1 chopped garlic or organic garlic powder

½ cup water

Salt and pepper to taste

Put catsup on top (try to find a kind with no corn syrup). I like jalapenos in mine. Add any other veggies that you like.

Put all ingredients into crock pot and mix well. Cover and turn on. Cook on low 3-4 hours or high 2-3 hours. This should make at least 4 meals.

To make a neat variety to this, cut the top out of large bell peppers and seed them. Add the uncooked meat mixture to the inside of the peppers. Top with catsup and place in crock pot. Cook the same as the meat loaf. Voila! Stuffed peppers.

Vegetable Lentil Soup

4 cups of dried lentils

32 ounces of any broth (organic no MSG)

2 cups water

1 onion chopped

The equivalent of 4 cups of any variety of vegetables, frozen or fresh that you like (Ideas: carrots, peas, lima beans, green beans, celery, squash, sweet potato)

28 oz. can diced tomatoes

4-6 cloves of minced garlic or organic garlic powder

Salt and pepper to taste

Place all ingredients in 5+ quart crock pot (if your crock pot is smaller halve this recipe.)

Cook on low for 7-8 hours or until vegetables are tender.

Hamburgers

Ground meat

1 t organic onion

1 t organic garlic powder

Salt and pepper

(I add turmeric too. Try it for a health boost.)

There are several different small appliances that will make a hamburger, even the crock pot. Mix all ingredients. Pat out to desired size and cook in desired small appliance. Gather fresh ingredients to put on top and pass on the bread.

Eggs With A Health Boost

2 eggs

Salt and pepper to taste

Shake on some turmeric

(Add a little at first, then the next time add more and so on until you can get the most possible on your eggs. Turmeric is a super spice. It is a huge boost for your health. Add it to everything you can.)

You can prepare this plain or add some onions and peppers or jalapeno peppers to spice it up a bit.

Scrambled or fried

You can use just about any means of cooking with eggs. The crock pot even works.

Hawaiian Chicken

2 pounds of cut up chicken

1 can of pineapple chunks in 100% juice

1 onion

1 bell pepper

4 T honey

Salt/pepper

Combine ingredients and cook on low for 8 hours in the crock pot or adjust to the cooker of choice.

Turkey Meatballs
with spaghetti squash

This is easy, but if you could make up the meatballs with sauce ahead of time it would make it even easier.

Meat balls

1 pound of ground meat

1 onion

1 t ground rosemary or herb of choice

1 T Italian seasoning

Mix and roll into balls

Spaghetti squash – Cut spaghetti squash in half. Take out seeds. Place cut sides down into crock pot or cooker of choice. Put meatballs on and around squash. Cook on high for 3 hours; check for doneness. When squash is done take it out and scrape out the "spaghetti" and place it in a separate bowl. Add a healthy ingredient spaghetti sauce to the pot with meatballs and warm on high until desired temperature. Spoon mixture onto spaghetti squash. *This should make at least 4 meals. Buy a small squash and halve the other ingredients if your cooker of choice is smaller, or if you don't need as much food.*

Beef and Broccoli

1 pound thinly sliced beef

1 cup organic (no MSG) beef broth

3 cloves of garlic minced

1 T honey

1 bag of frozen broccoli florets

Place all ingredients except broccoli into crock pot. Cook covered on low for 5 hours. When done add broccoli; cook additional 30 minutes on high.

Chili

1 pound of cooked ground meat

1 can kidney beans

1 can pinto beans

1 can black beans

1 can tomato sauce

3 T chili powder

1 onion finely chopped

2 cloves of garlic minced

Salt and pepper to taste

Add all ingredients. Cook on low for 6-7 hours or high for 4 hours in crock pot or in cooker of choice until done.

Add jalapenos on top if desired.

Chipotle Chili

2 leftover, peeled and chopped sweet potatoes

2-3 cups organic non GMO broth

1 pound cooked ground meat

1 large can of chopped tomatoes

1 chopped onion

1 ½ cup chopped cauliflower

2 cloves garlic minced

2 chipotle peppers chopped

> *(If you can't find chipotle peppers, you can add a small can of green chilies instead; it won't be chipotle, but it will be good.)*

¼ t cumin

Salt and pepper to taste

Peel and cube sweet potatoes. Add all ingredients. Stir. Cook on high in crock pot for 3-4 hours, or in cooker of choice until done.

Burrito Bowl

Cooked ground meat seasoned with

1 t cumin

1 T chili powder

1 t onion powder

1 t garlic powder

Salt and pepper

Salsa - *homemade or bought (Check ingredients. There are a lot with good ingredients and a lot without.)*

Guacamole – *homemade or prepackaged*

1 can of refried beans warmed up *(Check ingredients. They should be beans, salt, water.)*

Salad greens

In a bowl, add ingredients in any order that you want. I usually put my salad greens on the bottom and work my way up to the meat last.

Baked Salmon

2 - 6 oz. Wild caught Alaskan salmon fillets

Thinly sliced lemons

1 cup sliced green onions

Coconut oil

Salt and pepper

Preheat toaster oven to 400 degrees.

Arrange salmon on greased (coconut oil) pan at 400 degrees. Bake for 14 minutes or until desired doneness.

Sauté onions in coconut oil until almost done, add lemon slices cook 2 minutes. Sprinkle onion mixture over fish with a little more salt.

Bean Soup

4 cloves minced garlic

1 onion chopped fine

½ pound carrots or bag of baby carrots

4 stalks of celery chopped fine

1 pound dry beans (white northern or navy) washed

1 t ground rosemary

½ t thyme

Salt and pepper

6 cups water

Add all ingredients. Cook on low 8 hours or high for 4 to 5 hours in the crock pot.

Shredded Chicken

2 pounds fresh boneless chicken *(If using frozen add to cook time.)*

1 t oregano

1 t onion powder

1 t garlic powder

1 cup organic chicken broth, *(non GMO no MSG) or you could use water and add more salt.*

Add all ingredients to crock pot and cook on high 3-4 hours or low 5-6 hours. Keep broth that is in the pot, add carrots, celery, and chicken to make soup.

Add BBQ sauce to the shredded chicken, for BBQ.

Put leftover or fresh salsa, chopped avocado, and beans over it. Use your imagination.

Salmon Salad

A can of wild caught salmon *(When you open it up it should be very bright salmon in color.)*

Add any or all of these:

Chopped pickles

Chopped celery

Chopped onions

Mayonnaise *(look for no soy mayo)*

Chopped egg

Mix together and serve on a romaine lettuce leaf or get the circle sliced carrots and use it as a dip.

Roasted Vegetables

Any or all of these vegetables

Broccoli

Squash

Cauliflower

Carrots

Onions

Garlic

Asparagus

Brussel sprouts

Sweet potatoes

Chop, cube or slice vegetables into bite size pieces. Place on roasting pan. Drizzle coconut oil over them. Add salt and pepper. In toaster oven or appliance of choice, roast at 350 degrees for about 30 minutes or until done. Check often.

Roast to BBQ

Cook a roast in the appliance of choice. **Day one:** eat as a roast with vegetables. **Day two:** shred, add BBQ sauce and have BBQ the next day.

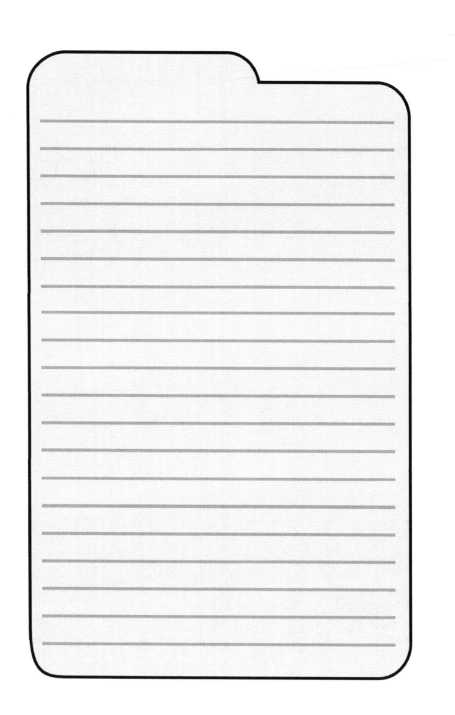

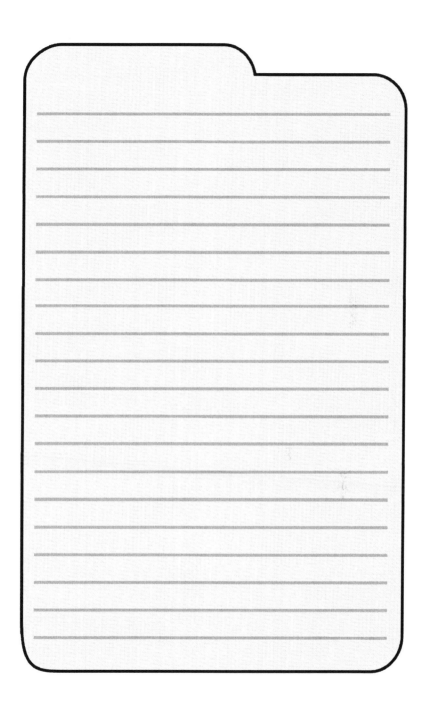

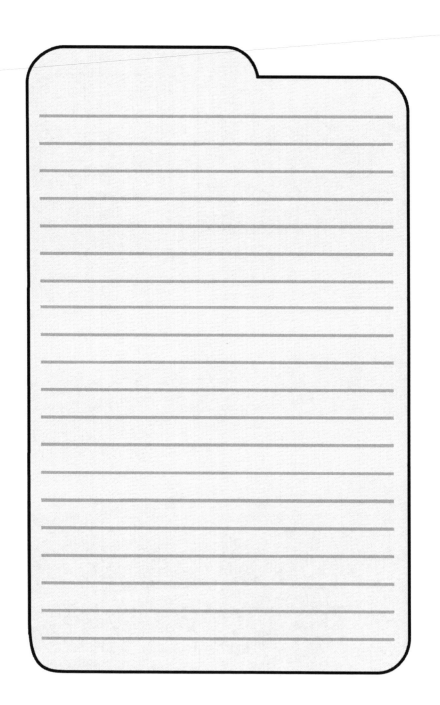

Keep in mind, many of the snacks in this book can be used as desserts.

Cinnamon Pecans

4 cups raw pecans

2 T coconut oil

4 T honey, maple syrup, or coconut sugar

2 T cinnamon

¼ t salt

Add all ingredients to crock pot and stir well. Cook for 3 ½ hours on low, stirring every 30 minutes or so.

Crock Pot Apple Dessert

4 diced apples *(You can also use pears for this dish.)*

1 t squeezed lemon

2 T honey, maple syrup, or coconut sugar

2 t cinnamon

½ t ground nutmeg

Cook on high for 2 hours or until very soft. If you have made the cinnamon pecans, crumble them on top to add even more yumminess.

Healthy Chocolate Shake

1 can of coconut milk *(Not the lite version)*

1 T cacao powder *(Healthy chocolate)*

Vanilla to taste

A pinch of salt

A natural sweetener to taste

Ice

Add these to make more shake or to add flavor

1 banana or 1 frozen banana

Almond or sunbutter

½ Avocado

Strawberries

Blueberries

Cherries

There are several ways that I have made this. Using a personal blender, add base ingredients first, then add any other ingredients. Blend.

Fast Fix For Chocolate

½ cup of unsweetened large coconut flakes
or 1 cup of a raw nut of your choice.

1 T cocoa powder (Cacao)

½ t organic coconut oil

1 ½ T honey or maple syrup

Melt the coconut oil (In the dash.)

Mix all ingredients together. Roll into balls
or eat with a spoon.

Avocado Chocolate Pudding

(Don't knock it till you try it!)

2 ripe avocados, peeled

1 ripe banana

1/2 cup cocoa powder (cacao)

A natural sweetener to taste

1/3 cup coconut milk

2 t vanilla

Blend all ingredients in a personal blender. Chill for 30 minutes. Eat!

⸺ Chia Pudding ⸺

I love this stuff!!! The sky's the limit on what you can do with this and it is SO healthy.

Banana Cream Pudding

1/2 cup coconut or almond milk

5 T white or black chia seeds

1 t vanilla extract

2 bananas

1 t lemon juice

pinch of cinnamon (optional)

In a personal blender, add everything except the chia and blend.

Add the chia, place a lid on the container, and shake well. Wait five minutes and shake well again. Do this several times. When desired consistency is met, it is done. *If you blend the chia in with the other ingredients, it will make the chia somewhat ground. There is nothing wrong with that; you might even like it better. Try it both ways.*

Chocolate Chia Pudding

1 ½ cups of coconut or almond milk

1/3 cup chia seeds

¼ cup cocoa (cacao) powder

2-5 T maple syrup, honey (to taste)

½ t cinnamon

¼ t salt

½ t vanilla extract

Blend all ingredients well in personal blender. Put in the fridge for at least 2-3 hours (If you can wait that long.) You can top with fruit or nuts if desired.

Strawberry Chia Pudding

3 T chia

1 cup of coconut or almond milk

1 T honey, maple syrup

1 t vanilla extract

2 cups fresh strawberries

In jar combine chia, milk, vanilla and sweetener. Put lid on it and shake VERY well. Refrigerate 4-5 hours. When done, puree strawberries in personal blender and add to the chia mixture to finish.

For some variety: Do the same thing but add fresh peaches, banana, blueberries, blackberries, raspberries, oranges, pineapple, mango, cantaloupe, lemon, lime, or even chopped nuts. These chia desserts are also good for breakfast. Yes, dessert for breakfast, YIPPEE!

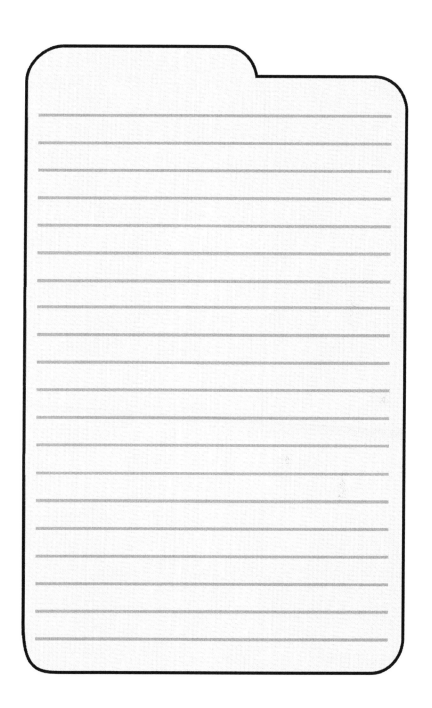

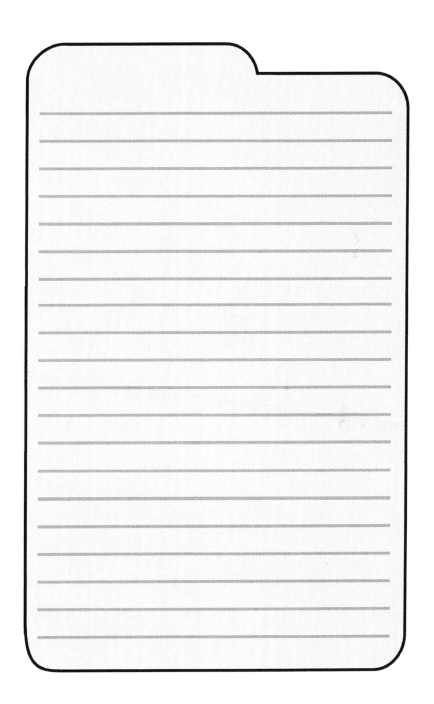

～ Conversion Chart ～

Unit:	Equals:	Also Equals:
1 tsp.	1/6 fl. oz	1/3 Tbsp.
1 Tbsp.	1/2 fl. oz	3 tsp.
1/8 cup	1 fl. oz	2 Tbsp.
1/4 cup	2 fl. oz	4 Tbsp.
1/3 cup	2¾ fl. oz	¼ cup plus 4 tsp.
1/2 cup	4 fl. oz	8 Tbsp.
1 cup	8 fl. oz	1/2 pint
1 pint	16 fl. oz	2 cups
1 quart	32 fl. oz	2 pints
1 liter	34 fl. oz	1 quart plus ¼ cup
1 gallon	128 fl. oz	4 quarts

Volume Conversions: Normally used for liquids only.	
Customary Quantity	**Metric Equivalent**
1 teaspoon	5 mL
1 tablespoon or 1/2 fluid ounce	15 mL
1 fluid ounce or 1/8 cup	30 mL
1/4 cup or 2 fluid ounces	60 mL
1/3 cup	80 mL
1/2 cup or 4 fluid ounces	120 mL
2/3 cup	160 mL
3/4 cup or 6 fluid ounces	180 mL
1 cup or 8 fluid ounces or half a pint	240 mL
1½ cups or 12 fluid ounces	350 mL
2 cups or 1 pint or 16 fluid ounces	475 mL
3 cups or 1½ pints	700 mL
4 cups or 2 pints or 1 quart	950 mL
4 quarts or 1 gallon	3.8 L

Note: In cases where higher precision is not justified, it may be convenient to round these conversions off as follows:

$$1 \text{ cup} = 250 \text{ mL}$$
$$1 \text{ pint} = 500 \text{ mL}$$
$$1 \text{ quart} = 1 \text{ L}$$
$$1 \text{ gallon} = 4 \text{ L}$$